## A Caregiver's Well-Being

"Caring for a loved one with dementia can be an isolating and overwhelming journey—but it doesn't have to be. This compassionate guide reminds caregivers they are not alone and empowers them to care for their loved ones while safeguarding their own well-being—a true lifeline in difficult times. Packed with practical suggestions and wisdom, this is a must-read road map for caregivers seeking guidance, reassurance, and hope even in the toughest moments."

—**Christine A. Padesky, PhD,** distinguished founding fellow, Academy of Cognitive & Behavioral Therapies; cofounder, Center for Cognitive Therapy; coauthor of *Mind Over Mood: Change How You Feel by Changing the Way You Think*

"This book would be one of the first resources I would use if I found myself needing to care for a person living with dementia. Tom and Donna Finn—both medical professionals—share their knowledge and their personal caregiving journey with Donna's mom. Caregiving is unfortunately known to be a lonely, stressful path, but the Finn's book is like a big hug and a deep breath, relieving the daily stresses while also finding a renewed relationship with those you care for."

—**Carrie Aalberts, MS,** also known as Dementia Darling, dementia advocate and educator; cohost of *Gather Darlings* podcast

"Admonition for self-care without providing rational understanding and concrete guidance compounds the stress and frustration of those who care for loved ones living with dementia. NOT *A Caregiver's Well-Being!* With the professional knowledge and skills of an experienced clinical psychologist and the wisdom and empathy forged in caring for a loved one, the Finns provide a gold mine of deep understanding and proven practical guidance for healthfully managing the inherent stress of caregiving. Even more, they guide caregivers on a journey toward psychological, relational, and spiritual wholeness as they care for those they love."

—**Bishop Kenneth L. Carder,** Ruth W. and A. Morris Williams, Jr. distinguished professor emeritus, Duke Divinity School; author of *Ministry with the Forgotten: Dementia Through a Spiritual Lens*

# A Caregiver's WELL-BEING

How to Master Stress and
Find Balance While Caring for
Loved Ones with Dementia

Thomas Finn, PhD
Donna Finn, PT, MS

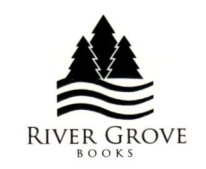

RIVER GROVE
BOOKS

This book is intended as a reference volume only, not as a medical manual. The information given here is designed to help you make informed decisions about your health. It is not intended as a substitute for any treatment that may have been prescribed by your doctor. If you suspect that you have a medical problem, you should seek competent medical help. You should not begin a new health regimen without first consulting a medical professional.

Published by River Grove Books
Austin, TX
www.rivergrovebooks.com

Copyright © 2025 Thomas Finn, PhD & Donna Finn, PT, MS

All rights reserved.

Thank you for purchasing an authorized edition of this book and for complying with copyright law. No part of this book may be reproduced, stored in a retrieval system, or transmitted by any means, electronic, mechanical, photocopying, recording, or otherwise, without written permission from the copyright holder.

Distributed by River Grove Books

Design and composition by Greenleaf Book Group and Jonathan Lewis
Cover design by Greenleaf Book Group and Jonathan Lewis
Cover images used under license from ©Adobestock.com/ icemanphotos; ©Pixabay.com/users/louanapires
Publisher's Cataloging-in-Publication data is available.

Print ISBN: 978-1-63299-931-3

eBook ISBN: 978-1-63299-932-0

First Edition

To care partners everywhere who are navigating the rip currents of dementia.

# Contents

**Preface**

**Chapter 1:** Care Partners and Stress . . . . . . . . . . . 1

## Section I Preparation: Know the Conditions

**Chapter 2** Know the Conditions: Symptoms and
Warning Signs of Dementia . . . . . . . . . . 17

**Chapter 3** Know the Conditions: Obtaining a Diagnosis . . . . . 29

**Chapter 4** Know the Conditions: Ongoing Health Care
and Support . . . . . . . . . . . . . . . . . 35

**Chapter 5** Know the Conditions: Legal, Estate,
and Financial Planning. . . . . . . . . . . . 39

**Chapter 6** Know the Conditions: The Patterns of
Our Relationships . . . . . . . . . . . . . 49

## Section II: Navigation—Skills for Managing Emotions

**Chapter 7** Don't Panic 1: Physical Domains of Coping . . . . . . 57

**Chapter 8:** Don't Panic 2: Psychological Domains of Coping . . . 71

**Chapter 9:** Yell for Help: Social Domains of Coping. . . . . . . 103

**Chapter 10** Keep Your Eyes on the Shore: Discovering Deeper
Meaning in Our Care Partner Relationships. . . . . 117

**Chapter 11** Swimming Sideways: Changing Our Care
Partner Behavior . . . . . . . . . . . . . . 133

**Chapter 12** Untangled but Knotted in Love . . . . . . . . . . 165

**Chapter 13** Epilogue . . . . . . . . . . . . . . . . . . 169

**Acknowledgments** . . . . . . . . . . . . . . . . . . . . . . 171
**Appendix:** Care Partner Resources . . . . . . . . . . . . . . . 173
**Notes** . . . . . . . . . . . . . . . . . . . . . . . . . . . . . 175
**Glossary.** . . . . . . . . . . . . . . . . . . . . . . . . . . . 181
**Index** . . . . . . . . . . . . . . . . . . . . . . . . . . . . 185
**About the Authors.** . . . . . . . . . . . . . . . . . . . . . 193

# Preface

A *Caregiver's Well-Being* provides a framework for managing the emotions we experience while caring for persons living with Alzheimer's disease or other forms of dementia. Whether you have been serving in a care partner role for years or, especially, if you are new to the emotional challenges that come with caring for someone with dementia, we hope to offer practical perspectives on caregiving that can build pathways to both improved coping and personal growth.

Written with the belief that good preparation for serving as a care partner is vital to our own well-being and for the well-being of those for whom we care, *A Caregiver's Well-Being* is conceptualized as a "primer" for working through the emotional, legal, medical, and social challenges of caregiving and targets how we can navigate these challenges in healthy ways. Realistically, becoming a "master" of caregiving stress never means removing emotions from our experience. Instead, mastering stress means developing the knowledge and skills necessary to effectively handle the anxiety, fear, frustration, sadness, and guilt that we feel as we try to meet the needs of a loved one who is living with a very difficult disease. In our own experience as caregivers, we are frequently told that we should manage stress but always benefit the most from people who show us how to do so. In the pages ahead, our goal is to provide such a *how* through proven psychological and behavioral tools that can lead to stress mastery, balance, and improved well-being.

We were very new to the stress of caregiving when Donna's mother began to show signs of cognitive decline in 2015. In many ways, this book is both a personal reflection on our experience of caring for Mom and a sharing of information that we have found immensely helpful in supporting her as she developed more significant signs of dementia. It has been an honor to walk with Mom on this journey, and we have been blessed with support from many people. We are grateful for the family, friends, support group members, and professionals who have offered us their time, prayers, and expertise. Our circle of support has grown and changed over the years, but always has been vital. Throughout this book, various resources for seeking support are mentioned, and they are summarized in the Appendix. They will be helpful in creating one's own circle of support so necessary for well-being as caregivers.

One caregiving challenge we should initially identify is related to the use of terminology found in the field of dementia. *Alzheimer's disease*, *dementia*, and *neurocognitive disorders* are terms often used interchangeably in today's caregiving circles. The Alzheimer's Association makes a useful distinction between the terms *dementia* and *Alzheimer's disease* that we will mirror in the chapters ahead:[1]

*Dementia* is an umbrella term for symptoms that are negatively impacting one's daily living activities. These symptoms can include problems like memory loss, language deficits, and issues with other cognitive capabilities, and can be attributed to many underlying conditions, illnesses, and other events. Alzheimer's disease is the most common cause of dementia symptoms.

*Neurocognitive disorders* is the general term that encompasses the varied symptoms of dementia. Neurocognitive disorders have specific categories that are named after their specific causes; these are the terms that most of us recognize and can include labels such as *neurocognitive disorder due to Alzheimer's disease* or *vascular neurocognitive disorder*. These formal-sounding titles are most commonly adapted in conversation to Alzheimer's disease or vascular dementia, so we will use these latter terms throughout this book. (We will look in depth at the issues of terminology in Chapter 2.)

Also, rather than use diagnostic labels that risk reducing a person to a diagnosis (e.g., "an Alzheimer's patient"), our preference is to use terminology that speaks about your loved one as "a person living with dementia," "a person with Alzheimer's disease," etc. This more accurately reflects our belief that all people possess an inherent dignity which defines their identity, and that they are not defined by their illnesses or loss of abilities. Also, while we will refer to statistics and research in the chapters ahead, we understand that each person's journey through dementia and caregiving is fully their own. Amid any generalization, we are aware that we are describing unique persons who are not simply numbers in a research study, but rather persons of infinite human worth whose dignity remains undiminished by their experiences and who are deserving of profound respect.

Another area of terminology seeks to describe people who provide support to those living with dementia as *caregivers* or *care partners*. Currently, we are in our eighth year of supporting Donna's mother on her journey of living with dementia and have used both terms in describing the ways we interact with Mom. Much has been written and discussed in professional circles about which is the better description, since labels can carry important meanings that shape expectations and behavior. Personally, we prefer *care partner* since it speaks, to us, of an exchange between people in which we both impact one another in meaningful ways. As partners, we give of ourselves and receive gifts from the other that enrich us and offer opportunity for each other's growth and well-being. Care partnering also aids in the recognition that we are part of a team that provides support to a loved one.

The term *caregiver* can sometimes imply a more one-directional relationship in which one person gives and one person receives, which can place the receiver in a passive role. Conversely, the term *care partner* calls each person to a mutual process that values shared decisions, problem-solving, troubleshooting, and communication, not just about physical health issues, but also about the thoughts and feelings we all experience. While it is this mutual care partner relationship that we value with our loved ones, we understand that many of us still use the terms *caregiver* and *caregiving*. When we use these terms, please be aware that we always envision this as a process reflecting the reciprocal connections that both bless and challenge our experiences together as care partners. The terms *caregiver* and *care partner* both begin with the word *care*, so let's begin to explore the mastery of stress and emotion as we care for our loved ones with dementia.

CHAPTER 1

# Care Partners and Stress

Most of us have been touched in some way by the realities of Alzheimer's disease or other forms of dementia. In our own lives, Donna's grandmother and Tom's mother lived their last years with dementias in various forms. Currently, Donna's mother is living with a mixed Alzheimer's and vascular dementia diagnosis in a nearby assisted-living community, and we are her closest family care partners.

On a broader scale, as of 2023, a tsunami of nearly 6.7 million people in the United States and 58 million people around the world are estimated to be experiencing dementia.[1] While this is often called the global "Dementia Crisis," most relevant to each of us are our own individual journeys of caregiving, which can be marked by waves of fear, sadness, anger, guilt, and pain that come when we suspect and finally confirm that a loved one has a diagnosis of dementia.

We remember the day this wave first hit, when Donna's mom received the diagnosis of mixed Alzheimer's and vascular dementia.

Working as a clinical psychologist (Tom) and a rehabilitation services manager in home health (Donna) did little to prepare us for the anxiety, sadness, frustration, and uncertainty that followed. Since that day, we have experienced the impact of such emotions through periods of reduced sleep, quick tempers, increased worry, and depressed moods that sometimes seem to materialize out of nowhere. These emotions are voiced through questions like "What is Mom going to need?", "How are we going to make this work?", and "What if she will need to be cared for in a facility of some kind?" Other emotions show themselves in the frustration of questions we've asked Mom, like "Don't you remember, I told you that yesterday?" or "Why would you think such a ridiculous thing?" It seems like our feelings keep getting tangled up in the tasks, demands, and responsibilities that our care partner roles require and, in turn, lead to feeling guilty when we realize that the more stressed out we become, the more stressed out Mom becomes, which sometimes causes her dementia symptoms to worsen. All of this makes us less effective in problem-solving the financial, legal, and medical tasks that need to be accomplished so that Mom can be safe and secure. Clearly, we have some serious untangling of emotions to do.

## Tangled

What do you think of when you hear the word *tangled*? We immediately envision our daughters as young children, when we would try to brush their tangles out while rushing around in the morning before elementary school. How those strands of hair could get so knotted up remains a mystery.

Although the specific causes for Alzheimer's disease and other dementias are not fully clear, brain research is making progress in identifying signs of the potential biological changes, or biomarkers, in our brains that play a role in the cause of dementia-related illnesses. We know that some conditions, such as Alzheimer's disease, involve a "tangling" of organic matter, called *tau proteins*, inside our brain cells that occurs as we get older.[2]

Since information is processed in our brains via the transmission of electrical or chemical impulses traveling among circuits of brain cells, these organic tangles in our brain circuitry can mirror our kids' hair tangles in a brush: Our brains' organic materials get twisted up and choke off nutrients that our brains need to maintain healthy brain cells. As a result, cells in various parts of our brains begin to die off, and the signs of their demise show up in symptoms such as loss of memory, confusion, and physical decline.[3]

All of this combines to make providing care to a loved one with dementia very stressful. Six out of ten care partners report that their stress levels are "high" to "very high."[4] As a result of such stress, we can begin to experience our own depression, anxiety, physical health problems, financial pressures, anger, and conflict in relationships with our loved one and other family members. Our stress becomes tangled with the love and care we try to provide to our loved ones, and we can feel very conflicted and "twisted up."

## Mastering the Stress of Caring

While scientists around the world are trying to solve the biological mysteries of protein tangles in Alzheimer's disease, we can focus on our personal experiences of stress and work to solve the mysteries of emotional tangles that twist our relationships with our loved ones into bundles of tension. Our hope, in the discussion that follows, is to target some of the underlying reasons that can make caring for people with dementia—and caring for ourselves—so emotionally difficult. With such an understanding, we can begin to build the concrete coping strategies necessary to better manage emotions in ways that lead to three major outcomes:

1. Improved psychological well-being.
2. Greater emotional consistency in relationships with your loved one.
3. The discovery of a deeper meaning in your care partner relationships.

As you work toward these outcomes, instead of remaining tangled in stress and tension, you can become more deeply knotted in love with your loved one.

## Why Is Caregiving So Stressful?

Learning that your loved one is experiencing dementia is like living through a natural disaster. In general, we humans prefer relatively predictable, secure surroundings that allow us to feel safe and balanced. When sudden, frightening experiences, like tornadoes, earthquakes, and wildfires, strike with little warning, our sense of security flies out the window and anxiety and stress come flying in. Our secure balance of life is replaced with feelings of vulnerability, insecurity, and stress. When the words *Alzheimer's disease* or *dementia* are first used to name your loved one's problems, the balance in life we had previously known flies out and uncertainty, fear, and stress fly in.

Reflecting on our own experience, the signs of Mom's developing dementia began seven or eight years before she was formally diagnosed with Alzheimer's disease and vascular dementia. After Donna's father died, Mom showed signs of increasing anxiety, difficulties with problem-solving, and narrowing in her social world. We didn't truly realize how bad this had become until we traveled with her and the rest of the family on a

Mississippi River riverboat trip celebrating her eighty-eighth birthday. This was the first time in a long time that she had to navigate sleeping away from home. The initial night of the trip involved a hotel stay in St. Louis, where she became very confused. She was unsure of where she was and what she needed to do to get herself ready for bed. Through her tears, we saw that she was frightened by what was happening to her, and the week on the riverboat required us to broadly problem-solve for her for the first time. In doing so, we felt a new level of stress as we tried to recreate a familiar structure like what she was used to at home, to cope with her growing cognitive challenges.

In the weeks following, we found ourselves thrust into caregiving at a level we had not expected Mom to require and felt shaken and unsure of what her actual needs might be. Seemingly without warning, life's balance was now out of whack. During the years since then, our caregiving stress has come in various waves, triggered by things like Mom's falls, illnesses, formal diagnosis, moves to higher levels of care, hallucinations, delusions, and most recently, her frequent inability to express herself coherently. In between these challenges, we are often hit with a realization that so many care partners share: We are losing her while she is still here with us. In addition, the desire to cherish the relationship we still have with her is often submerged under a tide of demands and tasks to be completed.

## Stress and You

Stress can be summed up as our brain and body's reaction when life events throw us off balance or disrupt our equilibrium. Stress impacts us on every level of who we are as a person. If we humans were pizzas, we'd be a pie of five slices or dimensions of personhood.

- Physical: Our bodies, with all the systems—nervous system, digestive system, circulatory system, respiratory system, endocrine system, etc.

- Emotional: Our feelings, like happiness, sadness, anger, fear, and guilt
- Psychological: Our thoughts, values, attitudes, and assumptions
- Social: Our relationships and interactions with our world
- Spiritual: Our relationship to God, the divine, a higher power, the universe, and the deeper meanings we find in life

Stress can disrupt how we function in any of these dimensions. When stress is particularly prolonged (as in care for someone with dementia), those disruptions can lead to significant dysfunctions, such as anxiety or depressive disorders. No matter how much the world likes to joke about keeping the "fun" in dysfunctional, that is difficult to do when walking as a care partner with a loved one.

## Stress and Your Brain's Fight-or-Flight Response

Understanding stress starts with understanding the brain and body's fight-or-flight response. These instincts for survival are hardwired into our nervous system and are triggered whenever we sense that we are threatened or vulnerable. When vulnerability and danger are perceived, a series of brain parts with odd names (like *amygdala*) send an emergency message to our hormone system that tells it to pump stress hormones like adrenaline, cortisol, and other compounds into our bloodstream. These stress hormones forward the alert message to important body parts that move them into survival mode by activating many physical and mental reactions.[5] For example, our

- Lungs breathe faster to get more energy-boosting oxygen into our body.
- Heart beats faster to move that oxygen to the big muscles of legs and arms.
- Pupils widen to improve vision.
- Stomach/digestion slows down, so we have more energy to run or fight off the threat.
- Muscles tighten up—especially in our abdomen—to create a "coat of armor" to protect important organs.
- Mind narrows its attention down to the specific threat and blocks out other distractions.

When our survival is actually being threatened (e.g., being chased by a big dog or taking shelter after a tornado warning), these reactions are extremely helpful and get us through the period of vulnerability in positive ways, such as running to safety. When the actual threat passes, our brain sends an "all clear" message to our body's various systems and soon, our liver and kidneys are draining all that adrenaline, cortisol, etc., out of our bloodstream and we feel back in balance.

## The Hurtful Impacts of Stress

But what if the threat doesn't pass? What if the stressor is one of ongoing uncertainty that doesn't let up and repeatedly sends us messages of vulnerability or helplessness? When this happens—as many of us can attest to in our care partnering years—our fight-or-flight system remains set on high, and we can experience hurtful physical, emotional, psychological, social, and spiritual impacts. (Sometimes, staying at heightened levels for a very long time can even lead to our fight-or-flight system beginning to shut down, resulting in a sense of feeling immobilized).

## Physical Impacts

- Erratic sleeping patterns
- Increased stomach acid, leading to nausea, constipation, or heartburn
- Decreased energy and increased fatigue
- Weakened immune system and increased susceptibility to illness
- Increased blood pressure
- Weight gain from the increased glucose that the body releases in an attempt to increase energy

## Emotional and Psychological Impacts

### Flight Symptoms

- Anxiety
- Worry
- Feeling overwhelmed
- Obsessive thoughts about a loved one
- Anticipation of negative outcomes
- "What if" questions
- Underestimating one's own ability to cope (e.g., "I can't take this anymore.")

### Fight Symptoms

- Anger
- Frustration
- Irritability
- Blaming

## Defeat Symptoms

If our fight-or-flight reactions aren't bringing us relief, we can view ourselves as helpless or powerless to improve our situation. As a result, we feel defeated and can experience:

- Grief.
- Sadness.
- Guilt.

Compared to the death of a loved one and the finality of that loss, walking with someone who has dementia is a series of losses on multiple levels of relationship. As the years of loss increase, our grief increases and we can become depressed, often losing interest in usual activities. Sometimes, we can begin to believe that the anxiety, anger, or helplessness we feel is intolerable and turn to alcohol, drugs, compulsive media watching, computer use, video games, etc., as a way of numbing out the pain that we feel. Sadly, these attempts to avoid our own pain only lead to worsening struggles.

## Social Impacts

Ongoing stress and repeated fight-or-flight responses may also begin to play out in our social behavior. Social changes can include:

- Boredom.
- Isolation and withdrawal from family or friends.
- Refusal to ask for help.
- Seeking constant reassurance.

### Spiritual Impacts

Finally, the stress of caregiving can contribute to difficulties in the way we try to make sense of life and find deeper levels of meaning in our experiences. Many of us will find challenges in our spiritual lives, including:

- Feeling angry with God or a higher power.
- Doubting the purpose of life.
- Losing the meaning once felt in your relationship with a loved one.
- Avoiding religious or spiritual practices and participation.

## The Struggle of Self-Care

As you read through the above list, odds are that you recognized yourself somewhere in those struggles . . . We sure do. Luckily, there is some good news. Even though caring for a loved one with dementia does involve demands that tax our mind, body, and spirit, we have the capacity to meet those demands and not only survive in our care partner role, but thrive in it. To thrive as a care partner, however, requires that we commit ourselves to basic principles that help us effectively find balance and master our stress.

As an example, the Alzheimer's Association publishes wonderful stress-management principles for care partners. The Association's publication "Take Care of Yourself"[6] lists ten suggestions for managing caregiver stress.

1. Take a break.
2. Seek out community resources.
3. Become an educated caregiver.

# Care Partners and Stress

4. Get help and find support.
5. Take care of your own health.
6. Manage your level of stress.
7. Accept changes as they occur.
8. Make legal and financial plans.
9. Know you're doing your best.
10. Visit your doctor regularly.

Here is the problem:
Most of us don't regularly do those things.
Here is the question:
Why don't most of us regularly do those things?
Here is the answer:

Because the uncertainty, anxiety, frustration, and stress of our care partner roles insert themselves into our previously predictable lifestyle and send fight-or-flight shock waves through our pizza of personhood. Those shock waves pull our slices apart as we are met with demands and expectations for which we are unprepared. In addition, caring for someone with dementia creates new tensions or intensifies old tensions in relationships with loved ones, and even with other family members. Ultimately, we can end up feeling helplessly caught in a very "disrupted equilibrium," which can prevent us from heeding even the best self-care advice. Even if our personality prior to this has been one of consistent coping, we will often feel caught in rip currents of stress and lose sight of healthier ways to meet our challenges.

## The Rip Current of Caregiving

We think the metaphor of a rip current is a very accurate description of our own experiences of caring for Donna's mother. A rip current is a phenomenon that occurs along ocean coastlines. It is an alley of water that moves away from the beach and out to sea. Most days, these "rips" are hardly noticeable, but sometimes, like on windy days, they can become so strong and fast that they are dangerous. On days like these, large waves storm the beach and, since all that water can't roll up any farther on the sand, the water creates its own pathway and cuts its way through the incoming waves back out to sea. The power and speed of this outward-bound water can pull a swimmer quickly away from the safety of the shore.

Growing up on the northern New Jersey seashore, near Sandy Hook, we can recall many times when swimmers got caught in rip currents because they didn't understand what was happening. They didn't know how to navigate the rip and, because of their disrupted equilibriums, they panicked and could have drowned if not for the lifeguards' quick actions.

Just like the Alzheimer's Association has "Take Care of Yourself" guidelines for managing the stress of caregiving, there are also guidelines for preparing for taking care of yourself and navigating the stress of actual rip currents. You may have seen signs posted on beaches that often include these tips for survival:

## Preparation

- Know the conditions.
- Be aware of the weather, wave patterns, warning flags, etc., to prevent trouble.

## Navigation

1. Don't panic.
   Stay calm, ride with the flow until it slows down, and don't try to swim against it.

2. Yell for help.
   Let others know you're in trouble and in need of support.

3. Keep your eyes on the shore.
   Keep the beach in sight at all times to prevent becoming confused and disoriented.

4. Swim sideways, then angle toward the shore.
   Instead of trying to swim against the rip current, swim across it then toward the beach, riding the waves in as you go.

These rip current survival steps mirror the steps that we must take in preparing for and mastering the challenges of caring for a loved one with dementia. The chapters that follow will explore each step and identify the knowledge, tools, and strategies that will be useful in managing our emotions and realizing the outcomes we hope for: improving personal well-being, increasing consistency in our relationships with our loved ones, and discovering deeper meaning in our care partnering relationships.

# SECTION I

# Preparation: Know the Conditions

Mastering stress in any situation begins with good preparation and knowledge. The more we know about what lies ahead, the more prepared we can be for meeting challenges that come our way. Entering a care partner relationship with a loved one who has dementia is one such challenge best met through good preparation.

Looking back on the beginnings of caring for Donna's mother, we wish we had a better awareness and foundation in five areas:

1. The symptoms and warning signs of Alzheimer's disease and other dementias.
2. The steps involved in obtaining a diagnosis.

3. The ways to identify and obtain good dementia-related health care.
4. The estate-planning documents needed to help access medical care and provide legal and financial protections for persons living with dementia.
5. The impact that past relationship experiences and family dynamics have on intensifying the stress of serving as a care partner.

Similar to checking conditions like weather, tides, surf conditions, locations of lifeguards, etc., in preparation for going to the beach, having a preparation mindset puts us in the best position to cope with care partnering rip currents when they develop.

CHAPTER 2

# Know the Conditions: Symptoms and Warning Signs of Dementia

When we first see problematic signs of aging in our loved ones, it can be confusing and difficult to understand. As a person ages, it is normal to see changes in psychological abilities that are observed through various behavior changes. These psychological abilities are often referred to as *cognitive skills* and they are grouped into what are called *cognitive domains*.[1] In general, there are six cognitive domains:

- Complex attention: Focusing on tasks, concentrating while filtering out distractions, calculating things in our minds, etc.
- Executive functions: Making plans and decisions, flexibly shifting mental gears, being organized, etc.
- Learning and memory: Remembering recent and past experiences, retaining information, and using it to guide actions in the future, etc.

- Language: Expressing oneself in words, understanding others' words, labeling items, knowing a person's name, etc.

- Perceptual-motor: Perceiving experiences correctly, having good hand-eye coordination, awareness of places, using basic tools, etc.

- Social cognition: Recognizing one's own emotions, empathizing with other people's emotions, recognizing social cues, filtering language, controlling impulses, etc.

## Spotting the Signs

At the seashore, colored flags are used to tell us about weather conditions. There could be yellow flags, red flags, purple flags, combination flags, etc., and each would be a source of helpful information to guide your decisions on how to deal with what's happening that day at the beach. The symptoms of dementia are like those beach flags: If we know what to look for and understand what certain signs/behaviors mean, they can guide our care decisions in ways that help to manage stress. While persons with dementia each have individual expressions of symptoms, common warning signs in the different cognitive domains exist and can include the following:

- Complex attention:
  » Distraction
  » Shortened attention span
  » Reduced concentration and focus
  » Longer times needed to process information and/or complete tasks
- Executive functions:

# Know the Conditions: Symptoms and Warning Signs of Dementia

  - » Confusion
  - » Disorganization
  - » Lack of planning
  - » Difficulty moving from one task to another
- Learning and memory:
  - » Reduced short-term and long-term memory (long-term memory is often more intact at early stages)
  - » Increased frequency of making lists, writing down dates, keeping items in certain places, needing reminders
  - » Forgetting names or where items were placed
  - » Repeating statements or questions without recall of previous conversations
- Language:
  - » Difficulties in saying or understanding words and sentences (also called expressive or receptive aphasia, respectively)
  - » Trouble finding the correct words for items or the names of recognizable people
  - » Difficulties with concrete expressions of ideas, shorter sentences, etc.
  - » Substituting descriptions for specific items or people (e.g., "That flat, round cooking thing" instead of "frying pan")
- Perceptual-motor:
  - » Difficulty making sense of what is seen, heard, etc., and describing it to others
  - » Confusion about one's location
  - » Getting lost or frequent mid-activity forgetfulness
  - » Needing more time to do familiar tasks or hobbies

- Social cognition:
  - » Changes in social or emotional behavior
  - » Invading others' space, lack of safety awareness
  - » Withdrawal and isolation from friends
  - » Inappropriate statements, humor, criticisms, or topics of discussion (loss of a "filter")
  - » Reduced empathy toward others or lack of emotional regulation (quickly shifting from one feeling state to another)

There are many detailed resources, with varied examples, that describe the way warning signs and symptoms develop,[2] and taking time to expand your knowledge in this area is a solid step in building a strong stress-management foundation.

Over the course of several years, Donna's mother gradually began to demonstrate occasional changes in her cognitive skills, especially with memory, word finding, increased anxiety, and social withdrawal, but we never connected these as precursors of a developing dementia. That changed one day, while driving Mom to a restaurant. She was in the front passenger seat and began talking about Donna in the third person with no awareness that Donna was sitting in the backseat of the car. It was this experience that alerted us that Mom's situation was moving beyond mild decline and that something needed to be done . . . but what? Luckily, Donna had contacts through her work in home health care who, along with a wonderful local resource called the Center for Healthy Aging, advised us that connecting Mom with a gerontology specialist and obtaining a formal diagnosis of her symptoms was an important first step in developing a care plan. They were able to guide us in connecting with a physician who had a specialty in dementia care. This physician diagnosed Mom with mixed dementia: Alzheimer's disease and vascular dementia. We worried about how Mom would react to receiving this information, but surprisingly, she seemed relieved to have an explanation for her struggles and said, "Thank goodness . . . I thought I was going crazy."

## Terminology

As we age, it is normal to experience subtle, small changes in our memory, thinking skills, etc., that do not interfere with our day-to-day activities. This has often been referred to as *age-related mild cognitive impairment* (or mild cognitive decline). If such changes progress to the point that declines in one or more of the above cognitive domains impact a person's day-to-day abilities to function, then that person is said to be experiencing dementia. In the past, *dementia* referred to neurological declines primarily in the elderly. Today, in an attempt to broaden clinical understanding, various categories of dementia are grouped under a label called *neurocognitive disorders*.[3] If a person who is experiencing significant cognitive declines can still independently cope by making adaptations in basic routines or habits (like cooking simpler meals, writing lists, or taking medications regularly using a pill box organizer), then the declines are labeled *mild neurocognitive disorder*. If the declines, however, move to levels that interfere with a person's ability to maintain independence in daily activities and result in the need for significant assistance, then the declines are labeled as *major neurocognitive disorder*.

These labels are thought of as a spectrum and are designed to be broad in scope. Neurocognitive disorders include cognitive problems that result from causes like brain trauma or substance abuse, which are different from the gradual deterioration and decline in brain health usually associated with dementia. While this terminology is especially useful in areas of research and treatment of persons with these conditions, these newer terms can still be confusing. One care partner, for example, when told that her husband was diagnosed with major neurocognitive disorder, replied, "But I figured he had dementia." Since the terms *major and mild neurocognitive disorder* can still be a bit of a mouthful, the more familiar word *dementia* is still widely used in caregiving circles. When we use the term *dementia*, we are using it interchangeably with *neurocognitive disorder*, with a focus on symptoms that appear over time and gradually increase as a person gets older.

Just as *dementia* is a familiar word to many of us, we are also familiar with another common term: *Alzheimer's*. A common assumption is that Alzheimer's and dementia are the same thing. We didn't realize that all dementias are not Alzheimer's disease and that there are many categories, or subtypes, of dementia (aka neurocognitive disorders).

## Types of Dementia

Consider this comparison: If you learned that a relative was diagnosed with cancer, what would be one of your first questions? Ours would be, "What type of cancer?" This question would be based on the knowledge that cancer has different causes, symptoms, treatments, and, most of all, expectations. With an illness like cancer, knowing the exact condition and stage of progression helps us to create individualized care partner plans. Similarly, with the condition of dementia, our ability to create an individualized care partner plan will also benefit from knowing the specific subtype (condition) that our loved ones are experiencing, along with its probable stage. This is why obtaining a formal diagnosis is such a critical step.

The subtypes of dementia vary in how their symptoms develop and in the ways they impact our brains, cognitive domains, and behavior. Some subtype names are based on the underlying causes of exhibited symptoms, while others are simply named based on the type of symptoms. Be aware that there are fine lines between some of the categories, as they share many features. Also, many people are diagnosed with more than one subtype, which include the following categories as described in the *Diagnostic and Statistical Manual of Mental Disorders (DSM-V)*:[4]

Dementia (or neurocognitive disorder), due to:

- Alzheimer's disease
- Vascular disease (or cerebrovascular disease[5])
- Lewy body disease
- Frontotemporal lobe degeneration
- Parkinson's disease
- Mixed dementia ("multiple etiologies")

Officially, diagnostic categories of dementia would be worded this way: Major or minor neurocognitive disorder due to_____. In the blank will go a name like one of the conditions listed above. For Mom, the dementia she is experiencing is diagnosed as major neurocognitive disorder due to mixed dementia: Alzheimer's disease and vascular disease.

That wording is very technical, so remember that it's OK if we don't refer to the exact name of a loved one's condition in perfect medical-speak. That said, let's look at the major types of dementia.

## Dementia Due to Alzheimer's Disease

Dementia due to Alzheimer's disease is the most common dementia diagnosis (at least 60 percent).[6] The typical course of Alzheimer's disease is one of gradual and increasing declines in a loved one's memory and their ability to learn new information. Problems in other cognitive domains also increase over time, including depression, anxiety, poor communication, language issues such as word finding, and poor judgment. Key in diagnosing a person with Alzheimer's disease is the gradual nature of how a person's symptoms appear and worsen. Usually, there are not extended periods of time when symptoms level off (called *plateaus*).

The underlying causes for Alzheimer's disease appear related to changes in brain cell proteins that lead to the buildup of substances called beta-amyloid plaque and tau tangles that contribute to the gradual dying off of brain cells. The gradual worsening of symptoms reflects the gradual damage that these plaques and tangles inflict on the brain cells themselves. The exact causes of these changes are still being studied, but it does appear that genetic mutations play a role.[7]

## Dementia Due to Vascular Disease

*Vascular* refers to how blood flows through our body. Our heart pumps blood through our arteries to deliver oxygen and nutrients to the body's cells and then carts away waste through our veins. Brain injury or other blood-flow problems in our brain disrupt the rhythm of this process, and our brain becomes deprived of oxygen and nutrients. As a result, brain cells begin to die.

Dementia due to vascular disease is diagnosed in people when declines in cognitive domains are related to signs of problems in blood flow through the brain. These cerebrovascular problems can come in the form of strokes, ministrokes (temporary ischemic attacks, or TIAs), stenosis of the carotid arteries, cerebral aneurysms, etc. The type of symptoms that a person will show are usually related to where in their brain the damage occurs, since different brain areas handle different cognitive domains. With this type of dementia, difficulties in the complex attention domain such as reduced attention span and information processing speed are common. Problems with executive functioning such as confusion, disorganization, and troubles with multitasking are also frequent. Memory is impacted if cerebrovascular problems occur in the areas of the brain important to memory functions. When the impact to the brain is in an area responsible for movements, changes in your loved one's ability to walk and keep balance can occur.[8]

Dementia due to vascular disease often has a gradual onset, but more sudden escalations in symptoms can happen, likely due to new blood-flow disruptions in your loved one's brain. Symptoms can often plateau during periods when blood flow is more stabilized. This form of dementia commonly appears with other subtypes of dementia. Typically, no more than 10 percent of people with dementia are diagnosed with only vascular causes for their symptoms.[9]

## Dementia Due to Frontotemporal Lobe Degeneration

Our brains have many different layers, structures, and connections. If you looked at a map of the outside layer of our brains (called the *cerebrum* or *cerebral cortex*), you could identify different regions that are in the front (i.e., behind your forehead), in the back, on the top, and on the sides. The top is the *parietal lobe*, the back is the *occipital lobe*, the front is the *frontal lobe*, and the sides are the *temporal lobe*(s). It is the latter two regions—frontal and temporal lobes—that are impacted in the frontotemporal lobe subtype of dementia. Genetic and other biological factors seem to contribute to deteriorations in your loved one's frontal lobe (which handles many of our cognitive skills) and the temporal lobe (which handles language skills). In the early stages of the disease, typical symptoms show up as thinking, behavioral, and language difficulties. Behaviorally, your loved one will begin demonstrating declines in the cognitive domains of social cognition and executive functions. They may begin to show personality changes such as apathy and withdrawal or increased agitation, impulsivity, and socially inappropriate actions. They can also become rigid and exhibit repetitive, compulsive types of behavior. Language changes include difficulties with speech, comprehension, and word finding. Curiously, people with frontotemporal lobe dementia have fewer difficulties with learning and memory, at least in earlier stages.[10]

Overall, this subtype accounts for about 5 percent of overall dementia cases, and a very high percentage of people who begin to show symptoms before their 60s are eventually diagnosed with frontotemporal lobe dementia.[11]

## Dementia with Lewy Bodies

Lewy bodies occur in our brain's cerebral cortex when a type of protein becomes abnormally bunched or clumped together. These clumps can then lead to gradual declines, such as inconsistent attention span and lack of alertness. Other symptoms often include problems with sleep and the presence of visual hallucinations. Another component of dementia with Lewy bodies is the appearance of motor difficulties following cognitive declines that are like those seen in Parkinson's disease and cause challenges to one's walking, eating, etc. The sequence is reversed in actual Parkinson's disease, with the physical movement symptoms appearing before cognitive declines. For a loved one with dementia with Lewy bodies, problems with learning and memory do not typically appear until later in the disease. Approximately 5 percent of people with dementia are diagnosed with dementia with Lewy bodies.[12] This condition is also known as Lewy body disease or Lewy body dementia.

## Dementia Due to Parkinson's Disease

Parkinson's disease is a nervous system disorder that affects a person's physical movements, causing problems with walking and coordination. The cause is related to the clumping of the same protein that is involved in Lewy body dementia but in a different part of the brain. As mentioned above, the cognitive declines that a loved one experiences in this subtype occur after the physical problems of Parkinson's have already set in. Cognitive problems develop gradually and often include personality changes, emotional disturbances, hallucinations, and delusions (false beliefs that won't change in the face of evidence that proves the beliefs to be incorrect). The majority of people with Parkinson's appear to develop dementia symptoms especially in the later stages of the disease.[13]

## Other Subtypes of Dementia

Dementia symptoms can also be related to a number of other conditions. These include traumatic brain injuries, HIV infection, Huntington's disease, Prion disease, and other medical conditions. When dementia symptoms develop due to more than one cause, the term "mixed dementia" may be used. Mixed dementia can also be referred to as "dementia due to multiple etiologies" (that is, multiple causes). This is understandable due to the cumulative, often interacting factors that cause brain cells to deteriorate and die, such as vascular problems, oxygen reductions, protein abnormalities, etc.[14] Donna's mom, for example, was diagnosed with mixed dementia (Alzheimer's disease and vascular dementia) in her late 80s.

### Delirium

Another condition that is important to be aware of is *delirium*.[15] This refers to a sudden onset of difficulties in awareness, thinking, behavior, or emotions. Hallucinations or incoherent speech are possible, and the person is often alert but unable to concentrate and communicate coherently. A loved one can become restless and agitated or withdrawn and lethargic. While these symptoms might appear similar to dementia symptoms, their rapid appearance or faster escalation is often due to illnesses or other medical-related issues such as dehydration, decreased electrolytes, infections (e.g., urinary tract infections), medication problems, etc. Very different from dementia, delirium can appear within hours, can fluctuate while lasting for days or weeks, and is reversible. Delirium can occur in loved ones who also have dementia, so a thorough assessment should be conducted by their health-care providers to identify why delirium symptoms have appeared and what can be done to treat them.

At this point, you may be experiencing information overload, but remember that it isn't necessary to get tangled up in exact labels. Rather, if we have basic knowledge of the signs and symptoms of dementia, we will be in a better position to create a plan of care for our loved ones. As the years progress, it is likely that we will need to enlist many types of help and support as part of that plan. Just like it is good to know where the lifeguards are at the beach, we will benefit from knowing where to find good dementia support services.

# CHAPTER 3

# Know the Conditions: Obtaining a Diagnosis

As Mom's signs and symptoms of dementia became more apparent, the second area that we realized we were unaware of as new care partners was how to access support. At that point, a colleague of Donna's advised that we start putting together a dementia-skilled Care Team. This evolving Care Team would ultimately consist of health-care providers who not only could diagnose Mom's condition, but could provide the ongoing services that she would need to thrive to the best of her abilities. As care partners, we strive to advocate for a holistic view of our loved ones and seek out health-care providers who will treat them as whole persons, not simply a set of symptoms.

Most often, developing this Care Team starts with your loved one's primary care physician, or PCP. Although situations vary, PCPs often have the best current medical knowledge of your loved one's health, developed in a context of an ongoing relationship over the years. Some care partners are already in a pattern of meeting with a loved one's PCP, which helps to ensure that accurate information is being communicated.

Others are only beginning to participate in a loved one's care in this way. As you prepare to meet with your loved one's PCP, it is always helpful to have the following information written down:

**Current health and functioning.** Provide symptom descriptions using the cognitive domains as a guideline. Describe the timeline for when problems such as memory loss, confusion, language changes, problem-solving difficulties, etc., appeared or became worse. Be sure to describe any substance abuse or mental health issues along with cognitive or behavioral symptoms. Include descriptions of any trouble with daily living skills such as cooking, personal hygiene, driving, money management, etc. The more concrete examples the better.

**Current medications.** Write down all medications (prescription and over the counter), vitamins, supplements, etc., that your loved one uses and have copies of this list ready to leave with health-care providers. Be sure to note any side effects and time of day when medications are taken, as medication timing can sometimes play a role in a loved one's difficulties.

**Past medical history.** Assessing your loved one's current health often occurs in the context of medical history. Have a written list of medical issues such as diseases, heart attacks or strokes, blood pressure problems, infections, diabetes, falls, injuries, concussions, etc. Your loved one's family medical history should also be included, especially regarding relatives who have had dementia symptoms or diagnoses such as Alzheimer's disease. Psychological, social, and cultural issues are also important in providing a holistic picture of who your loved one is as a person.

An initial meeting will include talking about these topics but also will try to begin identifying possible causes of your loved one's symptoms. A review of body systems will usually include breathing, hearing, walking and balance, vision, heart health, etc., to see if there may be any physical problems contributing to a loved one's decline. If you haven't accompanied your loved one to previous appointments, don't be surprised to learn of medical issues that your loved one has kept secret. Also, be sure that your loved one has listed you as a permitted contact on health information privacy release forms. This is especially important as your loved one's condition progresses.

While PCPs can provide very competent care, some do not have specialized training and experience in care of the elderly and, more importantly, in the assessment and treatment of people with dementia. In situations such as these, it is important to seek out other professionals with eldercare and dementia care experience. Often, the PCP may refer you to another professional who has a geriatric specialty or to a multidisciplinary geriatric assessment center. Although we may not need an official referral to see other eldercare professionals, it is always good if the PCP can recommend a colleague in the field, as this helps with communication between health-care providers. There is a range of professionals to whom referrals may be made, including:

**Specialties in the care of older adults:**

- Geriatrician: A physician.
- Geriatric nurse practitioner: A registered nurse.
- Gerontologist: A professional caregiver (nonphysician) who provides nonmedical care.
- Geriatric psychiatrist: A licensed physician with a specialty in treating emotional and behavioral disorders in the elderly who can prescribe psychiatric medications.
- Geropsychologist: A licensed psychologist who provides psychological evaluations and psychotherapy to the elderly.

**Specialties in the care of all adults, not only that of older adults:**

- Neurologist: A physician who specializes in diagnosing and treating brain/nervous system conditions.
- Neuropsychologist: A licensed psychologist specializing in the way the brain and nervous system impact behavior. They conduct neuropsychological evaluations that help identify the severity of cognitive domain declines.

In our personal experience, we were able to have Donna's mother evaluated by a local geriatrician who was very skilled in the diagnosis of dementia. This physician was able to connect warmly and professionally with Mom and utilize various methods of assessing Mom's status, including different types of cognitive tests.

# Tests Used in Diagnosing Dementia

Another component of the diagnostic process used by many health-care providers is the use of varied testing tools. Since dementia cannot be definitively diagnosed through any one test, it is common for several different tests to be conducted. Such tests can include:

## Cognitive Tests

A cognitive test assesses thinking skills in areas like reasoning, attention, memory, perception, and language. These mental capabilities can be informally assessed during conversation in which the professional explores different areas, including whether individuals can state the day, date, and time; recall a series of numbers or words; perform mental computations; or describe current events. Cognitive skills can also be evaluated by one or more formal testing instruments that the professional administers either in person or in a computerized format. Some of these formal tests or screening instruments are:

- Mini-Mental State Exam (MMSE).
- Mini-Cog.
- General Practitioner Assessment of Cognition (GPCOG).
- St. Louis University Mental Status Test (SLUMS).
- Montreal Cognitive Assessment (MOCA).

## Laboratory Tests

Blood tests can be administered to rule out underlying medical problems that may be causing your loved one's symptoms. As scientific research continues, more physiological indicators of dementia, called *biomarkers*, are being identified, and some lab tests can shed light on issues like brain protein abnormalities. Evidence for problems like inflammation or infection can also be explored.

## Neurological Tests

Tests that assess the physical structure and functioning of the brain are often used in attempting accurate diagnoses of what is causing your loved one's condition. These tests can identify if there is physical deterioration in parts of the brain or whether there is evidence of tumors, protein abnormalities, recent strokes, or past bleeding. Other tests assess electrical and functional brain activity. Tests are chosen based on the type of information that is sought and include:

- Computed tomography (CT) scans.
- Magnetic resonance imaging (MRI) scans.
- Functional magnetic resonance imaging (fMRI) scans.

- Positron emission tomography (PET) scans.
- Electroencephalogram (EEG).

## Mental Health Tests

Evaluation of your loved one's mental health is also vital, as conditions like depression and anxiety can contribute to difficulties in cognitive skills and behavioral patterns. These assessments can be conducted by psychologists, psychiatrists, clinical social workers, and other mental health professionals and often include interviews with family members.

## Genetic Tests

Genetic research has found that some genes can cause or increase the risk for Alzheimer's disease. As of this time, many questions remain concerning specific gene interactions, and these tests are not yet part of the routine assessment process for dementia-related conditions.

# CHAPTER 4

# Know the Conditions: Ongoing Health Care and Support

After Mom's geriatrician had diagnosed her condition, both she and the office's geriatric nurse practitioner were then able to provide ongoing care and consultation as part of Mom's Care Team. They helped us develop a third area of knowledge we needed as caregivers: how to obtain ongoing health care and support services for her in the years ahead.

Prior to Mom's increased struggles, she had lived in an eldercare community that offered a continuum of living options and services. She originally lived there in a house with Donna's father. After his death, she had become increasingly isolated and had difficulties navigating the environment in and around the house, such as walking across the parking lot to get her mail. As a result, she moved into an independent apartment in another section of the community; she was living there when she was evaluated by the geriatrician.

After we became aware that dementia was at the root of her struggles, we had many discussions with Mom, our family, and her health-care professionals. These discussions addressed questions related to her safety, independence, and ability to perform the daily activities that had previously allowed her to successfully live on her own. Driving, grocery shopping, personal hygiene, going alone to physician appointments, etc., became topics of greater exploration as we were all now aware that she would require more assistance as the years progressed. Many questions needed to be answered, like:

- Is she safe living on her own?
- What kind of supervision will she need?
- How long should she keep driving?

Information obtained through questions like these guides us toward identifying the members of our loved one's Care Team. A wide range of helpful information is available for guidance in putting together a personalized Care Team, depending on the status of a loved one's condition and the available resources near you. Excellent sources of finding support include the Alzheimer's Association's Community Resource Finder[1] and the Administration for Community Living's Eldercare Locator.[2] Other sources for finding needed support can include your physician, local senior center, or family and friends who have experience in providing care for their own loved ones with dementia.

When it becomes apparent that your loved one cannot safely provide for their own self-care and other aspects of independence, a new set of decisions will follow that focus on providing more supervised care. You may try to provide initial levels of extra care in your loved one's home or you may decide to move your loved one into your own home. Often, the inclusion of support services during in-home care will help you make the time necessary for your own self-care. This type of support can include services from homemaker and companion agencies, licensed home health-care agencies, or adult day care programs. Providers such as occupational therapists can evaluate a loved one's current abilities and help guide decisions about creating a safe home environment. Some organizations also provide respite care that can last up to several weeks and allow for care partners to take time away and recharge their caregiving energies.

Your loved one's response to these kinds of services can range from gratitude to outright resistance, making it hard to find the best way to provide needed support. We've heard many creative ideas for easing these adjustments from professionals, friends, and support group members, including keeping initial visits short, describing new care partners as friends instead of "agency personnel," etc. The key is adapting your explanations to a context that is relatable and acceptable to your loved one and allowing plenty of time for the acceptance/adjustment process.

Another crossroad you may face is when your loved one's medical, cognitive, and behavioral declines intensify to the point that you are no longer confident you can provide for their safety and well-being at home. This is often a time of heightened anxiety and guilt, especially if you've made a promise to them that you would always keep them "at home, no matter what." A promise like this is always made from deep love and concern, but there are some circumstances where it isn't possible to maintain at-home care. It is at these times that some form of residential care begins to be considered, such as assisted-living or skilled nursing facilities. If you pursue this step, it is important to search for facilities that have expertise in care for persons with dementia. In addition to the above resources, here is a short list of other resources for ongoing care and support:

- Alzheimer's Association Community Resource Finder: https://www.communityresourcefinder.org/
- National Association for Home Care and Hospice: https://mynahc.nahc.org/directories/agency-locator?reload=timezone

- Medicare locator for home health services: https://www.medicare.gov/care-compare/?redirect=true&providerType=HomeHealth
- Administration for Community Living Eldercare Locator: https://eldercare.acl.gov/Public/Index.aspx
- Meals on Wheels America: https://www.mealsonwheelsamerica.org/
- National Adult Day Services Association: https://www.nadsa.org/locator/
- National Respite Network and Resource Center: https://archrespite.org/caregiver-resources/respitelocator/

# CHAPTER 5

# Know the Conditions: Legal, Estate, and Financial Planning

Having access to and detailed knowledge of your loved one's legal and financial status is the next prerequisite for managing stress as caregivers. We thought we were prepared for these areas when Mom's dementia symptoms began to appear. We had access to her financial accounts and knew that she had written a will, created advance directives, designated a power of attorney, etc. What we didn't realize was that these documents were quite old and had not kept up with current state laws. Even more importantly, the way that these documents had identified Donna and her siblings as coagents with power of attorney, estate coexecutors, and co-health-care agents had not accounted for demographic changes within the family that would complicate the fulfillment of these roles when needed. Finally, Donna's parents had set up a family trust with her mother as trustee, but this was a function that Donna's mother could no longer perform, given her cognitive decline.

Two nonfamily backup trustees had also been appointed, but one had long since retired and the other had died. Rectifying all of this created significant stress and required months of work to straighten out.

To avoid this kind of legally related stress, it is vital to have clear knowledge of a loved one's *current* legal and financial situation. Conversations about these matters can be difficult, particularly when paranoid thinking is a dementia symptom that your loved one is experiencing. Regardless of your situation, you cannot leave anything to assumption and must be sure that the steps and processes within the estate plan are clear and practical. We found many publications and websites that offer advice on how to navigate toward successful planning,[1] and we strongly recommend consulting a local eldercare attorney to be sure that you know the local and state requirements that need to be met. Below are important questions concerning six major estate planning topics:

- Finances
- Last will and testament
- Power of attorney
- Advance directives and health-care agent
- Do-not-resuscitate orders
- Conservatorship

These questions are formatted as worksheets to help you assess your loved one's current legal and financial situation as well as plan for their future needs. After each question, decide if you need to take action and, if so, circle "yes." We encourage you to consider these questions early in your care partner role and revisit them as your loved one's condition changes.

# Legal and Financial Assessment

## Finances

| QUESTION | IS ACTION NEEDED? | FIRST STEP TO TAKE |
|---|---|---|
| Should I be more involved in monitoring my loved one's finances? | Yes | |
| Should I reduce my loved one's risk for being scammed via the phone, email, direct mail, etc.? | Yes | |
| Should my loved one still have credit/debit cards? Is a credit freeze necessary? | Yes | |
| Should I add my name as a joint account owner or be approved as a cosigner on bank accounts? | Yes | |
| Do I need to help with or take over bill paying? | Yes | |
| Should I set up accounts for paperless billing or automatic payments? | Yes | |
| Should I get utility companies, banks, credit card companies, etc., to set up third-party notifications and contact me in case of late payments or unusual account activity? | Yes | |
| Do I have an up-to-date list of assets such as checking and savings accounts, investments, property, etc.? | Yes | |
| Do I have account numbers, usernames, passwords, PINs, etc., for these assets in a secure location? | Yes | |
| Should we reduce the number of bank or other financial accounts to help simplify finances? | Yes | |
| Are there other caregivers who should have copies and/or access to my loved one's financial information? | Yes | |
| If my loved one is resistant to changing/simplifying financial matters, will it help if we meet together with an accountant, financial advisor, or other professional? | Yes | |
| Have I communicated my/our desire to help my loved one with financial management in a way that reflects my concern rather than a desire for control? | Yes | |
| Are there any other financial issues that I should address? | Yes | |
| Do I need to become authorized to access my loved one's safe deposit box or post office box? | Yes | |

# Last Will and Testament

| QUESTION | IS ACTION NEEDED? | FIRST STEP TO TAKE |
|---|---|---|
| Does my loved one have a last will and testament that states how assets and personal property will be distributed after death? Are beneficiaries clearly identified? | Yes | |
| Do I know where to find my loved one's last will and testament (original copy)? Have I recently read it? Is it signed and are witnesses identified? Are copies of it with appropriate attorneys and relatives? | Yes | |
| Does the will address all my loved one's *current* estate planning desires and needs? | Yes | |
| Does the will identify an executor who will manage my loved one's estate and carry out the will's terms and instructions? | Yes | |
| Has a successor(s) to the executor been identified in case the executor is unable or unwilling to fulfill his or her role? | Yes | |
| Have the executor and successor executor expressly agreed to take on these responsibilities? | Yes | |
| Are there any challenges to the executor/successor(s) fulfilling their roles (e.g., geographical distance, conflicts of interest, conflicts of relationships, etc.)? | Yes | |
| If coexecutors have been identified and joint actions are required, will this create logistic challenges to the will's execution? If so, should the will be changed to a single executor or to state the coexecutors' ability to act separately? | Yes | |
| Have my loved one and I discussed funeral plans? Are these plans written down in a separate document or part of the will? | Yes | |
| Do we need to formally conduct pre-funeral planning with the funeral home of my loved one's choice? | Yes | |
| Are there any other last will and testament issues that I should address? | Yes | |

# Power of Attorney

| QUESTION | IS ACTION NEEDED? | FIRST STEP TO TAKE |
|---|---|---|
| If my loved one loses the physical or mental capacity to manage legal and financial matters, has someone been legally identified to act as an agent with power of attorney? | Yes | |
| Is the agent with power of attorney "durable," with broad access rights lasting until my loved one's death? | Yes | |
| Is the power of attorney document signed, and does it conform to local legal standards? | Yes | |
| Are copies of the power of attorney with appropriate attorneys and relatives? | Yes | |
| Has a successor agent with power of attorney(s) been identified? | Yes | |
| Are there any challenges to the agent(s) with power of attorney/successor(s) fulfilling their roles (e.g., geographical distance, conflicts of interest, conflicts of relationships, etc.)? | Yes | |
| If coexecutors have been identified and joint actions are required, will this create logistic challenges to the will's execution? If so, should a single agent with power of attorney be named or the coagents with power of attorneys be allowed to act separately? | Yes | |
| Since a copy of the power of attorney may not be the only document or procedure that a given company requires, do I need to check that the designated agent with power of attorney has *confirmed* his/her authorization to conduct business as my loved one's representative with: | | |
| Medicare and Medicaid? | Yes | |
| Veterans Administration? | Yes | |
| Social Security? | Yes | |
| Internal Revenue Service? | Yes | |
| All government and tax authorities? | Yes | |
| Insurance companies: life, health, disability, and long-term care? | Yes | |
| Banks and investment companies? | Yes | |
| Accountants, lawyers, and financial advisors? | Yes | |
| Physicians and other health-care providers? | Yes | |
| Phone, cable, and internet companies? | Yes | |
| Utilities (electric, gas, water, etc.)? | Yes | |
| Real estate brokers? | Yes | |
| Funeral homes? | Yes | |

# Advance Directives and Health-Care Agent (or Attorney-in-Fact for Health-Care Decisions)

| QUESTION | IS ACTION NEEDED? | FIRST STEP TO TAKE |
|---|---|---|
| Do I know my loved one's advance directives or other preferences regarding end-of-life care, including the potential for extraordinary care measures and do-not-resuscitate orders? | Yes | |
| Are these advance directives written and have they been discussed openly with all family members? | Yes | |
| If my loved one loses the physical or mental capacity to make personal health care decisions, has someone been legally identified to act as health-care agent to make health-related decisions, including decisions about life-sustaining treatments, organ/tissue donation, and releasing medical records? | Yes | |
| Does the health-care agent have access to my loved one's medical records, including lists of current medications and health-care providers? | Yes | |
| Is the health-care agent document signed, and does it conform to local legal standards? | Yes | |
| Has a successor health-care agent(s) been identified? | Yes | |
| Are copies of the health-care agent document with appropriate attorneys and relatives? | Yes | |
| Is the health-care agent document on file with necessary health-care providers or relevant agencies, including physicians, home health-care and hospice agencies, and assisted-living or skilled nursing facilities? | Yes | |
| Are there any challenges to the health-care agent/successor(s) fulfilling their roles (e.g., geographical distance, conflicts of interest, conflicts of relationships, etc.)? | Yes | |
| If co-health-care agents have been identified and joint actions are required, will this create logistic challenges in making health-care decisions? If so, should a single health-care agent be named, or the co-health-care agents be allowed to act separately? | Yes | |

# Do-Not-Resuscitate (DNR)/Do-Not-Intubate (DNI) Orders

| QUESTION | IS ACTION NEEDED? | FIRST STEP TO TAKE |
|---|---|---|
| In case my loved one's heart or breathing should stop, does he or she want CPR or other procedures to be performed for resuscitation? | Yes | |
| In case my loved one's heart or breathing should stop, does he or she want intubation (artificial respiration) to be performed? | Yes | |
| Is the DNR order included in the written advance directive? | Yes | |

# Conservator/Guardian

Another legal decision to consider is the identification of a conservator, sometimes called a legal guardian. While the duties of a conservator mirror many of the duties of an agent with power of attorney, there are distinct differences, including when the role of conservator takes effect (i.e., only after one is incapacitated), how it takes effect (by court order), and whether it applies to conservatorship of the estate, the person's day-to-day life, or both. Questions concerning conservatorship include:

| QUESTION | IS ACTION NEEDED? | FIRST STEP TO TAKE |
|---|---|---|
| If my loved one becomes fully incapacitated, has someone been legally designated to act as conservator? | Yes | |
| Is the conservatorship document signed, and does it conform to local legal standards? | Yes | |
| Are separate copies of the designation of conservator required or is the designation part of another document such as the assignment of the health-care agent? Are copies with appropriate relatives and attorneys? | Yes | |

*continued*

| | |
|---|---|
| Has a successor conservator been identified? | Yes |
| Are there any challenges to the conservator/successor(s) fulfilling their roles (e.g., geographical distance, conflicts of interest, conflicts of relationships, etc.)? | Yes |
| If coconservators have been identified and joint actions are required, will this create logistical challenges in making conservator decisions? If so, should a single conservator be named, or the coconservators be allowed to act separately? | Yes |

## Let's Talk About It

Even though talking with loved ones about aging, finances, and end-of-life issues is not a comfortable topic, the stress of talking about it will be reduced if we express our desire to be more involved with a tone of compassion and respect instead of fear, frustration, and control. It is difficult for loved ones to experience a loss of independence and autonomy. Since legal/financial topics are strongly tied to their sense of self-esteem and competence, focus less on telling them what to do and more on asking what they would prefer. In our conversations with Mom, we tried to use the principle of "ask first, give my opinion second." Questions like "How are you feeling about the way your bill paying is going?" seemed to result in better outcomes compared to leading with "I think I should start paying your bills." Mom experienced a good deal of stress whenever she believed we were telling her she was wrong about a certain issue, so leading with gentle questions typically resulted in better discussions. As it became evident that Mom was having trouble with finances, Donna asked, "It seems like there are a lot of checks to write lately. Would it help if I come over once a week and do them *with* you?" Mom was open to this and when she began to have trouble even paying bills with Donna, she again was open when Donna asked, "Writing all of these seems harder for you lately. How about I write out the checks and bring them over for you to sign?"

In sum, the process of addressing legal, estate, and financial planning matters helps reduce stress the most if we plan early, lead with compassion, stay flexible, reassess often, and always act with the best interests of our loved one at heart.

CHAPTER 6

# Know the Conditions: The Patterns of Our Relationships

The first four conditions we've discussed relate to concrete aspects of caring for a loved one. Signs and symptoms, diagnoses, health-care services, and financial and legal decisions are tangible factors that we address in ways that lead to practical outcomes. Next, let's look at a less concrete condition of caregiving: the history of our emotional relationship with our loved one. Our goal is to develop awareness of how old roles and patterns of relationships can surface during our care partner activities and produce unexpected stress.

Since childhood, Donna's mom had leaned on Donna for care and support. Donna's education and career as a health-care provider further established Donna in Mom's eyes as her primary physical and mental health problem-solver. As Donna began to accept an increasing role in caring for Mom, her stress increased. Stress stemmed from the time demands that were required and from occasions when Mom's words or actions triggered Donna's memories of difficult past experiences in their relationship. Those triggers caused powerful anger, sadness, and guilt. While we learn early as care partners that dementia may sometimes intensify a dementia sufferer's difficult personality traits, we have often been surprised to find that caring for someone with dementia can also intensify the historical relationship dynamics between loved one and care partner. Given this reality, there are significant benefits to knowing the emotional condition of our relationship with our loved one and anticipating these kinds of emotional triggers as we lean into our care partner roles.

There are many ways we can understand and conceptualize how our relationship experiences impact the ways we think, feel, and behave. Most perspectives of human development recognize that how we develop our personalities can be influenced by what happens over time between us and our parents, guardians, siblings, extended family, friends, peers, mentors, acquaintances, etc. Our self-esteem, personality style, emotional reactions, and stress-management skills flow from an interaction between nature and nurture. The genetic temperament we inherited from our parents is shaped by the lifelong experiences we have with those parents and all the people named above. At the point when our care partner role begins, all that history is ready to interact with the demands we are asked to meet. The greater awareness we have of such history, the better we will be at managing the challenges that lie before us.

One of the schools of thought that has been most helpful to us is the area of psychological theory and practice known as a cognitive behavioral perspective.[1] Cognitive behavioral principles look at the role that our thinking styles play in our feelings and behavior. We'll discuss this more in upcoming sections, but an important concept that relates to knowing the condition of our relationships is the concept of core beliefs or core fears. Made popular over recent decades by psychologists such as Dr. Judith Beck[2] and Dr. Jeffrey Young,[3] *core beliefs* refers to messages that we receive through our experiences in life that tell us about the "core" of who we are. In our minds, these beliefs can be heard as "I am" statements that define some aspect of our identity as a person. Hopefully, the messages we receive from life experiences are affirming and validating, such as:

"I am good."

"I am competent."

"I am secure and safe."

"I am loveable and significant."

Unfortunately, many of us receive messages that are invalidating, such as:

"I am bad."

"I'm incompetent and a failure."

"I'm weak and helpless."

"I am unlovable and unimportant."

The latter beliefs can act as fight-or-flight triggers, which cause unpleasant physical and emotional stress reactions. Since we are wired to survive and want to find ways of reducing stress, we learn to create our own emotional and behavioral coping strategies for calming or avoiding the difficult feelings that flow from hurtful core beliefs. Such rules for survival and soothing may help us feel better in the moment, but as we get older they just pull us back into similar riptides of stress and emotion.

Tom, for example, grew up in a New Jersey town where he was the youngest of his neighborhood friends and the only one with red hair and freckles. The teasing and bullying that he experienced contributed to the development of core beliefs of inadequacy and vulnerability. Those experiences were woven into other difficult family dynamics that reinforced similar core themes and led to a lot of internal stress and insecurity. To manage those feelings and reduce the tension, he developed behavioral and personality patterns of being quiet, shy, seeking acceptance, and avoiding criticism. Those patterns sometimes worked in the short run to avoid unpleasant emotions but only led to increased anxiety as the years moved forward, since his avoidant style prevented his learning more effective coping styles.

Donna's family experiences, while generally loving, stable and secure, included those caregiving components with her mom that we mentioned above. As Mom experienced medical/psychological issues, like bad headaches related to anxiety, Donna would often be assigned the role of "looking out" for Mom, which sometimes included sleeping on Mom's bedroom floor if Donna's dad was away. Over the years, Donna felt pressure to continue that role so she could avoid core fears such as "I'm not being good enough" or "I'm bad" and reduce feelings of guilt and sadness.

As Mom's dementia progressed, she became critical of Donna's caregiving. During one instance, Mom was very angry at Donna, chastising her for never visiting her—even though Donna had visited the day before. Old core messages of "not good enough" were loudly amplified in these interactions, and Donna was again challenged to work through the resulting guilt and frustration. Talk about rip currents!

To explore our own conditions of relationship with our loved one, we invite you to answer the following "Rip Currents of Dementia" questions. This is a series of questions we've found helpful in anticipating the emotional triggers that can complicate our care partner roles. It takes time to explore these themes, and it is possible that such exploration may elicit difficult emotions. In some situations, especially if your relationship history with your loved one involves significant pain, we encourage you to seek help through dementia support groups or personal counseling.

# "Rip Current" of Dementia Questions: Core Triggers of Stress

## Core Messages

- What direct or indirect messages about myself did I receive from my loved one during my youth, teens, and adulthood?
- Did my experiences with my loved one send me messages that I am bad or incompetent? How?
- Did my experiences with my loved one tell me that I am not good enough or unimportant? How?
- In my relationship with my loved one, do I feel: Inadequate? Vulnerable? Weak? Like a failure? Invisible? Insignificant? Like a disappointment?

## Roles

- What has my role with my loved one been like over the years?
- How did my loved one expect me to act when it came to:
  - » Fixing problems?
  - » Reducing or avoiding difficult emotions?
  - » Their own feelings of loneliness?
- In what ways am I still expected to fulfill these roles?

## Painful Themes

- Are there any unresolved painful or difficult themes in my relationship with my loved one?
- Was my loved one controlling or dependent? Is there a history of abuse or excessive criticism?

- Did I ever feel neglected?
- Did my loved one compare me negatively to others?

As you consider these questions, it would be ideal if your answers reflected a history of experiences full of affirmation, support, validation, and unconditional love. Unfortunately, pain is often more memorable than joy. If your relationships included difficult experiences through which you perceived messages of invalidation, hurt, and conditional love, you will benefit from building skills that prevent your loved one's current behavior from aggravating old core wounds. How to do so is challenging and takes time, so we will focus on this specifically in Chapter 8. For now, knowledge that these patterns can exist is crucial for mastering stress and finding balance in your care partner roles, especially when you place this knowledge into context with the other medical, financial, and legal strategies to form a blueprint for the successful management of caregiving stress. Hopefully, these chapters have helped you consider how well prepared you are for the stress that lies ahead. Having looked at these areas of preparation, let's next look at how you can develop skills for coping with the emotions you experience as part of your care partner role.

SECTION II

# Navigation: Skills for Managing Emotions

Do you know the most common reason that swimmers require rescue? Most lifeguards will give a very consistent answer: "The swimmers were in over their heads." In lifeguard-speak, this means that the swimmers lacked the swimming skills needed to safely navigate the depth of the water or the currents swirling around them. As we've said, regarding our own care partner experiences, we were in over our heads as caring for Mom began to intensify. Luckily, in addition to improving the practical knowledge of the medical, financial, and legal aspects of dementia caregiving, what has helped us most to keep from "drowning" in stress has been learning to build skills for improving our own psychological well-being. Not only has that helped us emotionally, but it has led to developing more consistency in our care partner relationship with Mom. The chapters that follow focus on ways to build stress-management and relationship-consistency skills while targeting specific strategies for mastering emotions like anger, guilt, anxiety, and sadness that are so common when living as a care partner.

CHAPTER 7

# Don't Panic 1: Physical Domains of Coping

Earlier, we talked about beachside warning signs that list ways to survive ocean rip currents. Invariably, the first two words of advice on those signs are "Don't panic." We've often laughed at such a suggestion! Think of it: You're swimming in the ocean, when suddenly, you realize you are being pulled away from shore against your will and toward a seemingly endless ocean full of potentially nasty creatures, and the sign says "Don't panic"? Sorry to say, but most of us would panic! When being pulled out to sea, our brain's fight-or-flight reaction rejects the "don't panic" instruction and immediately injects adrenaline and other stress hormones into our bodies. With this stress hormone rush, we feel driven to swim straight back toward the beach, without realizing that this direct route is right into the rip current. If we do swim against the current, we quickly become exhausted by our efforts and are then at high risk of drowning.

Caregiving is full of similar emotional currents. Moments like learning of an initial dementia diagnosis or being unable to find a parent who disappears after driving to the grocery store create rushes of anger, anxiety, sadness, guilt, and frustration that pull us away from our shores of emotional comfort. At other times, more subtle emotional tides well up, like when a loved one forgets our birthday, or forgets something we just said, or when we first become aware of the gradual "loss of one who still lives." Experiences like these trigger fight-or-flight responses of varying intensity, and it's common to feel emotionally overwhelmed. A friend of ours was shocked when her husband was diagnosed with early onset Alzheimer's disease. Her husband had usually handled all household and money-related decisions, and within six months, she had to learn how to take over bill paying and long-term financial planning, as well as unfamiliar household chores and repairs—all while preparing to sell their home. It was very hard *not* to panic.

When faced with these kinds of stressors, is it truly possible to stay calm and cool and never feel overwhelmed or out of control? Frankly, no. The experiences of fear, anger, and sadness are a natural and normal reality of the care partner role. It is possible, however, to recognize our stress reactions and work our way through the physical, emotional, psychological, social, and spiritual rip currents of care partner stress before they pull us from shore. As we mentioned earlier, we humans are integrated beings of body, mind, and spirit. We can't react on just one dimension without the other dimensions being involved, so let's consider steps we can take to manage stress in body, mind, and spirit.

## Physical Domains of Coping

Initial signs of stress often first appear in our bodies. These physical signs can include muscle tension, sighing, fatigue, poor eating, reduced exercise, and trouble sleeping. Like many care partners we know, we began to experience such symptoms as the need to provide more care for Mom increased. Remember that stress will trigger these physical reactions because our fight-or-flight systems sense danger and want to protect us from perceived harm. In the face of these physical impacts, what can we do to cope more effectively on a bodily level?

## Gentle Breathing

The most direct way to calm our bodies is to breathe slowly and gently. Remember that stress results in more rapid and shallow breathing in an attempt to boost energy via increased oxygen. If we consciously slow the pace of our breathing, we can send a message to our brain that we are *not* in danger and can start to reduce the hyperventilation brought about by fight-or-flight reactions. There are many ways to control breathing,[1] and our personal go-to strategy includes these steps:

- Breathe in slowly through the nose as if trying to smell a favorite scent.
- Picture your lungs as balloons and try to fill them only half full. (Remember, when we're stressed, we have too much oxygen in our bodies already, so we don't want to become more hyperventilated.)
- Breathe in air gradually; don't force it in all at once.
- Breathe with your abdomen (belly), not with your chest.
- Pause after the inhale for a second or two.
- Breathe out slowly through the nose or mouth.
- Pause after the exhale for a second or two.
- Repeat.

It is difficult to teach ourselves to breathe slowly when we are in the heat of a stressful moment, so it's important to practice gentle breathing on a regular basis when we're not feeling stressed. Ideally, we could all take fifteen to twenty minutes twice a day to sit comfortably or lie down, close our eyes, and focus on breathing gently, but that is not easy to pull off. Our care partner lives are extremely busy, and breaks like that are hard to find. If that's your situation, take time to practice while watching TV, cleaning the house, cooking, grocery shopping, or sitting in traffic (minus the closed eyes, of course). There are also various computer or smartphone apps that are helpful in the practice of calm breathing.[2]

An additional breathing tool that we have found helpful is pairing a word or two with a gentle breathing pattern. While breathing slowly, saying a word like "calm" while exhaling allows our brain to pair the word with the more relaxed bodily state.[3] With enough practice, a calmer body can become conditioned to the repeated word, even amid a stressful moment.

## Senses for Safety

If fight-or-flight reactions are triggered by perceptions that we are not safe, then realizing that we actually *are* safe can help soften those reactions. In addition to gentle breathing, we can use other sensory pathways to reinforce that we are not in danger nor being threatened when difficult caregiving situations occur. Often referred to as anchoring or grounding tools,[4] these sensory strategies involve using our five senses to focus our attention on the present moment and gain a more objective perspective on what's happening.

For example, one man who was a care partner for his mother with Alzheimer's disease would frequently become angry with her when she would repeatedly ask him the same question every few minutes. Instead of continually snapping at her by saying, "Don't you remember you just asked me that!?" he taught himself to remain silent and apply what we might call the "Wisdom of Threes":

- Visually find three blue objects in the room.
- Touch and concentrate on three different textures.
- Tense and slowly release three different body muscles.

As he did each step, he became more aware that he and his mother were safe and, although he was dealing with deep sadness and frustration, he could stay calm even as she repeated her questions.

While one of the most common versions of this sensory-grounding technique is Dr. Ellen Hendriksen's "five sights, four textures, three sounds, two smells, one taste" technique,[5] the basic strategy in any version involves tuning into what you see, touch, hear, smell, and taste while allowing your mind to absorb the details of the present experience. For example, look around the space you are currently in and experience your own "Wisdom of Threes":

- Find three objects of a certain color. Describe to yourself what the objects are and how they are different or similar.
- Slowly touch three different textures. Describe those textures and how they feel to you.
- Listen for three different sounds. If it is completely quiet, listen to your breathing, or even to the sound of silence or the ringing in your ears. If necessary, create sounds by moving your hand or foot.

The more we practice using our senses to focus on the present moment, the more we can remain calm in care partner moments of stress and discomfort. As with breathing, the key is to practice these sensory focus exercises when we are not feeling high levels of stress so we are better prepared to apply them when stressful situations occur. It is especially helpful to practice gentle breathing exercises in conjunction with sensation focusing, as together they are powerful allies in stress reduction.

## Physical Movement and Exercise

Physical movement itself is a helpful stress-management tool. Slowly walking down the hallway, jogging in place, swinging our arms or legs, slowly clenching then releasing our fists, etc., are sources of reassurance for our brains that we are in control and not helpless in the midst of uncomfortable events happening around us.

Imagine a day when you are feeling anxious, frustrated, and stressed following a difficult interaction with your loved one. Picture that you enter the kitchen, about to make dinner for your family. You begin to notice a feeling of tension across your shoulders. Before pulling out the cooking utensils, you make a conscious decision to walk slowly out onto the porch and look around the yard for three minutes. As you do, you begin to breathe gently with your abdomen and focus your eyes on the yellow lilies and black-eyed Susans in the garden, noticing how they move in the afternoon breeze. Your hands are on the porch railing, and you move your fingers around it while tuning in to the texture of the railing and how it is constructed. You walk around the porch and listen for the sound of the birds chirping while feeling the breeze as it caresses your face and tousles your hair. Being present in such a moment via our senses is a wonderful "don't panic" gift to give ourselves, and it all started with walking from the kitchen to the porch!

We have also found that physical movement is often helpful in reducing Mom's stress and agitation, especially if we can encourage her to focus her senses on the surroundings of her neighborhood hallway and courtyard. Getting up and moving also helps her to interact with her neighbors and other care partners, which always helps ground her and reduce tension.

Getting regular physical exercise can be a difficult habit for care partners to begin and maintain. Most of us know the importance of exercise and are aware of the health guidelines that organizations like the Centers for Disease Control and Prevention recommend, like 2.5

hours a week of moderate exercise along with another two days a week of muscle-strengthening activity.[6] Regular exercise not only helps reduce stress but also reduces risks for most mental and physical health problems, including the development of dementia. Many of us just don't work exercise into our weekly routines, often citing reasons from what we call "The Lack List," a list of the various explanations we give ourselves for not moving. These include a lack of:

- Time ("I just don't have time.")
- Money ("I can't afford it.")
- Energy ("I'm just too tired.")
- Enjoyment ("I hate feeling sweaty or sore.")
- Knowledge ("I just don't know what to do or how to start.")
- Opportunity ("I can't find someone to watch the kids.")

Lack List reasons are real. Care partnering or other life events do make it hard to exercise regularly, so there is no need to feel guilty or inadequate when we get out of routine. While the obstacles of time, money, opportunity, etc., are relevant challenges, the root challenge is that many of us do not truly value physical exercise and activity in our lives. To *value* exercise means you believe enough in its importance to put that value into action. Valuing exercise means that you know it is so vital that you're willing to problem-solve your Lack List issues to figure out how to make exercise a part of your week-to-week lifestyle.

There is a big difference between a good idea and a value. Picture sitting in an auditorium with a hundred people. The leader of the group says, "If you think it is a good idea to exercise regularly as a component in a healthy lifestyle, please stand up." How many people would stand? Our guess is that over 90 percent of the people would stand up.

Next, the leader of the group says, "If, in the last week, you exercised for a minimum of 2.5 hours and did some strength training on at least two days, please remain standing. If you did not do all of that, please sit down." How many people do you think would still be standing? Our guess: fifteen to twenty-five, if we're lucky!

This illustrates the difference between a good idea and a value. Nearly all of us think exercise is a good idea. Not all of us, however, have transformed that idea into a value that drives our behavior toward making exercise part of a healthy self-care routine. Early on in caring for Mom, we were using a number of excuses on our own personal Lack List—time was short, energy was low, etc.—and we were not doing a very good job in the self-care department, especially with exercise. We realized that we had lost focus on the value we had usually placed on being active. In addition, we realized that to master the stress of being care partners for Mom, we had to recommit to making regular activity and exercise part of our weekly routine. It's also been highly motivating to know research shows that lack of exercise is a risk factor in developing both cardiac *and* cognitive disease!

There are countless sources for developing regular exercise routines. These are available from health-care providers, local libraries, the internet, etc. The key is to develop a plan that best fits your current physical condition and lifestyle realities. Whether it's walking around the neighborhood, yoga exercises in the basement, climbing stairs, riding a bike, or joining a gym, any first step will help start building momentum. If you need a place to start, try an internet search of "exercise for busy people." Most suggestions will focus on beginning with just five or ten minutes of activity creatively plugged into the routines of your day. Again, the key here is that your loved one will also benefit from your taking care of your body as best as you can.

## Sleep

When care partners get together, one of the more frequent questions we ask each other is, "How are you sleeping these days?" The most common answer is, "Not enough."

Although it is common that care partner demands result in an occasional bad night of sleep or two, another negative impact of ongoing stress is the way it interrupts our ability to sleep over an extended period of time. We tend to stay up too late, lie awake for long periods of time before falling asleep, wake up often during the night, and, generally, don't feel rested when we get up in the morning. Lack of sleep can be particularly problematic if caring for a loved one at home, especially if your loved one develops their own sleep problems. It's no surprise, then, that another important component of coping in the physical domain is developing healthy sleep patterns.

How to improve sleep is a well-researched area of self-care. In general, we know that if we reduce overall stress, we sleep better. Even when stress is high, however, there are many nonmedical steps to take for improving sleep quality. The first set of strategies for sleep improvement falls under the umbrella term of "sleep hygiene."[7] This refers to various actions we can take during the day and evening to give our brain and body its best shot at sleeping seven to eight hours at night. A typical list of sleep hygiene suggestions includes:

- Avoid watching video screens just before bed (thirty to sixty minutes minimum). Light from screens may reduce melatonin levels, which is a hormone necessary for good sleep.

- Go to bed and get up at similar times every day, regardless of whether it is a weekday or weekend and regardless of how well you slept the night before.

- Do not use your bed for anything other than sleep or sexual intimacy. This means no reading in bed, watching TV, etc.

- Don't nap during the day and, especially, no nodding off while watching evening TV or reading.
- Try to minimize stress in the evenings, including limiting media that can trigger worry or anger, such as TV news or suspenseful movies. (Limiting such media for your loved one is also important.)
- Keep bedrooms as cool and as dark as possible.
- Limit caffeine (from all sources), especially after 12 p.m.
- Don't eat too close to bedtime, and avoid alcohol and heavy snacks after dinner.

One care partner–related sleep hygiene topic to consider is preparing for late-night phone calls either from your loved one or from another member of the Care Team. In our personal situation, this has been an ongoing process of decision-making. As the course of Mom's dementia progressed, she lost awareness of time and would call Donna's cell phone in the middle of the night for many nonemergency reasons. There have also been other times when one of her facility caregivers has called following a fall or other health emergency that required Mom to be evaluated at the hospital emergency department.

Experiences like these obviously interfere with sleep and require us to make some difficult choices. Do we leave our phone ringers on or silence them overnight? Do we allow Mom to have a phone? Do we set up some type of "rotating call coverage" among family members? Do we utilize a landline/cell phone combination so that facility staff calls a certain one at night in case of emergency and we turn the other off? These are difficult questions, and it took several years of trial and error to arrive at a plan of keeping our cell phones in do-not-disturb mode overnight, knowing that Mom's facility would call our landline if there was an actual emergency. (Most cell phones also will ring in do-not-disturb mode if the number is dialed twice in a row.) This plan required working through the guilt that we felt for not answering a call from Mom late at night or early in the morning. We had to learn to trust that she was in a place where other competent care partners were looking out for her and that they would help her through whatever issue she was having at the time of her call.

If sleep-support strategies like these don't bring about enough improvement, there's another tool for improving sleep patterns called cognitive behavior therapy for insomnia, or CBT-I.[8] This tool focuses on the importance of our thought patterns, which we will discuss, but also involves changing our behavior after we get in bed. If we lie in bed awake with endless tossing, turning, and ruminating, we risk conditioning our brain to believe that lying in bed isn't for sleeping but rather for tossing, turning, and ruminating. In CBT-I, calm breathing and sensory strategies are often utilized to help us settle down for sleeping, but the important component is a significant behavior change: If you are not asleep within twenty minutes of your head hitting the pillow, then get out of bed and sit somewhere without much light or mind-awakening activities (no phones, etc.). A comfortable chair in the bedroom or nearby room is a good option for sitting and looking at nothing more exciting than a dull magazine. Sitting up and using some of the previously mentioned strategies, like breathing, sensory focusing, etc., combined are very helpful in calming our systems down enough to help our brains head toward Slumbertown. The goal is to relax enough so that you start to feel sleepy again. When you feel your eyes getting heavy or sleepiness beginning to return, go right back to bed. If you're still awake in another twenty minutes, repeat the process.

While this is certainly challenging, it has worked for us and many others who stick with it. Sometimes we don't get a ton of sleep the first night or two and feel very tired the next day. Should this be your experience, be sure you don't nap before going to bed the next night.

## Diet and Nutrition

The last aspect to discuss in the physical domain of stress coping is healthy eating. This is another area where we let items on our Lack List derail us from making healthy changes. Healthy eating guidelines are found in many places[9] and usually involve balanced nutrition patterns that target eating more food that is good for our hearts and brains (vegetables, fruits, healthy proteins, and fats, etc.) and fewer processed foods that contain high sugar, saturated fat, cholesterol, etc., which aren't good for our hearts and brains. While we know healthy foods benefit us, the realities of stress and limits on our time push us toward grab-and-go processed foods. Also, let's be honest: Foods with high sugar and fat taste good, and they make for quick stress relievers. There is a growing availability of healthy grab-and-go foods, but we have to seek them out.

On an emotional level, we've noticed that we eat worse when the stress of caring for Mom is high and we're feeling trapped, frustrated, helpless, and unable to pursue other life opportunities or activities. At these times, we don't feel in control of life and then, in a moment of semi-rebellion, take control of a certain junk food and put it in our mouths, feeling like we deserve to treat ourselves. In the end, however, we just feel less in control and the stress continues.

Although we've personally improved our diet and nutrition routines over the years, there are days when we still overeat the bad stuff, like handfuls of chocolate chips and bigger bowls of ice cream. We did find, however, that better planning is the key to improvement. Knowing what we want to eat, committing to shopping for it, and then taking time to prepare it (even ahead of time) has been a tremendous help. We've also learned to accept that we're not going to be perfect in our food choices, so being less judgmental of ourselves helps as well. Since so much recent research has revealed how eating a heart-healthy diet reduces bodily inflammation, improves our immune system, and even reduces risk for future dementia, it is extra clear why building healthy nutrition habits is a vital component of managing stress.

Should you be looking for a plan to start changing your eating style, make an appointment to talk with a health-care provider about what might work best given your starting point. Again, there are many good resources for improving nutrition as well as sources of support in various group settings or online programs. The key will always be finding a plan that works for you and then committing yourself to it. When it comes to eating, it does take time to create habit change so, if need be, start small. Maybe start with breakfast and make improvements in this meal for the first month. Next month, add lunch, and so on. Whatever small steps we can begin to take, we will be better for it!

CHAPTER 8

# Don't Panic 2: Psychological Domains of Coping

In addition to the ways stress can make us feel like we're in a battle with our bodies, it can also make us feel like we're in a battle with our minds. Serving as a care partner drops us repeatedly into wild rip currents of thoughts and feelings that produce waves of emotions like anxiety, anger, guilt, and sadness. Such waves are whipped up by thoughts that are worrisome, intrusive, and ruminating. Countless "what ifs" run through our heads as we anticipate the worst. We sometimes argue in our minds (if not in real time) with our loved one, family members, and health-care providers; and we can judge ourselves to be inadequate, unimportant, or helpless, all of which leaves us internally tangled in so many ways.

As challenging as all of this is, it is possible to master tools for reducing stress. In general, this involves two broad skill sets:

- Learning to develop more realistic and helpful patterns in our thinking styles.
- Learning to accept and flow with the stress we experience when we're not able to keep our thinking so realistic and helpful.

## Locus of Control

Many of the strategies for emotional and psychological coping are drawn from research and experience in the field of cognitive sciences and, in particular, the field of cognitive behavioral therapy, or CBT. An important concept in CBT is called locus of control,[1] which refers to how we explain the reasons why we experience things that happen to us. We can view our life circumstances as happening due to fate and forces outside of our control (external locus), or we can view ourselves as able to exert influence over life circumstances (internal locus). The concept of locus of control extends to our emotions, and we can explore where the cause, or control, of our feelings and reactions is located.

**External locus of emotional control** sees our feelings and their intensities as being caused by something that we can't control. From this perspective, the cause of our emotions can be something outside of us, like another person or situation, or it can be something inside of us, like a heart palpitation or other body symptom. With an external locus, we describe the feelings we experience as care partners with statements like:

- "She is making me so mad!"
- "This whole situation is driving me crazy!"
- "Losing him little by little is overwhelming me."
- "When I talk with her, I feel my chest tense up, and that sensation makes me so afraid."

**Internal locus of emotional control** is very different. It reflects how our feelings and reactions are multilayered products of our biological temperaments, body reactions, *and* the way that we think about our external circumstances and internal sensations. The term *thinking* refers to our mind's activities, such as the ideas, beliefs, attitudes, perspectives, perceptions, opinions, judgments, interpretations, assumptions, and projections through which we process and give meaning to our experiences. The meaning we give to our experiences helps bring the emotion forward. Although thoughts, feelings, and body reactions basically happen at the same time, we can understand how they operate if we analyze them in a sequence.

Here is one of our favorite illustrations of locus of control: You are driving home one afternoon and, up ahead, you see a kid running along the side of the road. As you drive by, the kid throws a brick at your car, smashing the windshield and putting a huge dent in your hood. How do you feel at that moment? An initial sense of shock, then anger? That would be our reaction. Now picture that you stop the car to yell at the kid but, suddenly, the kid yells to you, "Hey, please help me! My brother just fell off his bike and hit his head on the curb. He's knocked out and my phone is dead! Could you please call 911!?" You then see the unconscious brother lying on the side of the road. Now how do you feel? If you're like us, you'd end up less angry and feel more worried for the child. But why? What changes the intensity or type of feeling at the end of that scene? If our emotions were purely externally controlled ("The kid breaking my window made me mad"), our anger wouldn't change since, regardless of the eventual explanation, the throwing of the brick and its damage still happened. Most of us, however, don't feel the same anger, because the anger isn't simply a direct result of the brick. The initial anger is a product of an instinctive fight-or-flight response tangled in the thoughts we use to process the experience, such as *What an idiot! This shouldn't be happening. I can't stand kids like this, this is terrible!*

Let's consider this on another level. In reading the rock-throwing vignette, most of us probably pictured a boy throwing the rock even though the example just said that a "kid" threw the rock. This happens because, in an instant, our brain unconsciously projects meaning and interprets the event according to a stereotype that boys throw rocks at cars. A sense of danger is also instantly perceived that generates a rush of fight-or-flight adrenaline. When the kid informs us that we are not in danger but rather part of a crisis in which our help is needed, our mind shifts to an assumption that this is a kid in need instead of a rotten punk. This generates thoughts such as: *Oh no, this is an emergency, the brother might be dying. I wish the kid got my attention some other way, but I can deal with the car later. Now it's time to help.*

## Thought or Feeling?

To better understand how thoughts influence our feelings, it helps to recognize the difference between a thought and a feeling. People use the word *feeling* in many ways, but for this discussion, let's use it to refer to either a physical sensation or a pure emotional state at a given moment in time. When we ask ourselves *What am I feeling?* we could then answer with *I'm feeling* _____, where the word in the blank could refer to a physical sensation:

- *I feel muscle tightness in my arms.*
- *I feel pressure in my chest.*
- *I feel my heart beating really fast.*

We could also answer the *What am I feeling?* question with a word that refers to a specific emotion. Emotions fall into four broad feeling categories: happiness, sadness, anger, fear. (A fifth category of emotion called *disgust* is another basic emotion that captures how we can feel revulsion to specific things or behaviors that we find offensive. While this may come more into focus if our caregiving involves tending to our loved one's personal hygiene, let's focus mainly on happiness, sadness, anger, and fear that get tangled up in our stress reactions.) In this emotional dimension, *I'm feeling* _____ might be answered with:

- *I feel frustrated and angry.*
- *I'm feeling so sad.*
- *I'm feeling really stressed and anxious.*

If someone were to ask, "So, how are you feeling with how Mom is doing lately?" You might answer with a physical sensation: "I'm feeling so much tension in my neck and shoulders." You could also answer with an emotion: "I'm feeling just so sad." If you substitute a thought for an actual feeling such as "I'm feeling horrible" or "I'm feeling overwhelmed," it sets the stage for increased stress. Thoughts, as mentioned above, are those ideas, beliefs, attitudes, perspectives, perceptions, opinions, judgments, interpretations, etc., that give meaning to our experiences. Technically, words like *horrible* or *overwhelmed* are thoughts. They are interpretations or assessments of our circumstances or emotional states. Consider this example: Let's say your daughter's sports team won their big game last night and your friend asked, "Hey, how'd you feel about the game last night?" Which of the following answers identifies a feeling and which identifies a thought?

- **A.** "I felt like it was fabulous."
- **B.** "I felt so happy."

The feeling answer is B, as it speaks to a pure emotion while A is more of an opinion or thought about the game, even though it follows the words "I felt." Now try these and decide if the statement reflects a thought or a feeling:

1. "I feel this just shouldn't be happening."
2. "I'm so frustrated."
3. "I feel like I can't take this anymore."
4. "I feel . . . just so anxious."
5. "I feel depressed."
6. "She's driving me crazy."
7. "I'm so worried all the time."

(Answers: 1. Thought. 2. Feeling. 3. Thought. 4. Feeling. 5. Feeling. 6. Thought. 7. Feeling.)

In the normal flow of life, making this distinction may not matter, but when we are dealing with care partner stress and uncertainty, making this distinction will be very helpful in developing better stress-management skills. One tool for improving our ability to make the thought/feeling distinction and identify feelings more accurately is to create a basic "feelings vocabulary." Try this exercise:

Create a four-column grid on a piece of paper with the four emotional categories listed across the top and the numbers 1 through 4 (representing intensity of emotion) written vertically along the left side:

| Lowest | | HAPPINESS | SADNESS | ANGER | FEAR |
|---|---|---|---|---|---|
| | 1 | | | | |
| | 2 | | | | |
| | 3 | | | | |
| | 4 | | | | |
| Highest | | | | | |

Next, find words that label the increasing intensities of each emotion as you might experience them. You can come up with your own words or, if needed, look at a thesaurus or an internet synonym site for suggestions. Remember to look for words that are feelings and not thoughts. A feeling vocabulary grid might end up looking like this:

| Lowest |   | HAPPINESS | SADNESS | ANGER | FEAR |
|---|---|---|---|---|---|
|  | 1 | Content | Bummed | Ticked off | Uptight |
|  | 2 | Happy | Down | Annoyed | Worried |
|  | 3 | Joyful | Sad | Frustrated | Anxious |
|  | 4 | Ecstatic | Depressed | Enraged | Petrified |
| Highest |   |   |   |   |   |

Each of our individual grids will likely be different, and there is no right or wrong list. The key is to have words that allow us to communicate our emotions to others *and* to ourselves. It takes practice to build a working emotional vocabulary, and it can be helpful to write our feelings down in a journal. Taking time to write out our thoughts and feelings lets us "get them out," allowing for exploration and giving us a starting point for applying the tools and strategies that we will target in the next section. The more we are in touch with our emotions and have ways to process them, the less chance for stress to accumulate and interfere with life. There is, however, one major roadblock to success in doing this: Many of us are afraid to feel our feelings. We may fear the discomfort of intense emotions, or fear that feelings will overwhelm us, or believe that we are weak if we acknowledge difficult feelings. Ultimately, if we can allow ourselves to work through the short-term discomforts that unpleasant feelings bring, the long-term negative impacts of repressed or constrained emotions will be reduced. We recall reading to our children the book *The Hurt*, by Teddi Doleski, which is a very accurate description of this phenomenon.

## Coping Tools for the Mind

Caring for a loved one with dementia is a demanding, challenging, heart-heavy process through which we slowly lose the personal connection with someone who has held an important place in our lives. We cannot minimize the reality of how difficult and seemingly unfair this can be. Coping with this reality will be most effective if we embrace what we would call the "Resiliency Principle": The sadness, frustration, and pain that comes with being a care partner will be borne most resiliently if we can find a deeper meaning in the suffering before us. We were initially told about this by other experienced care partners, and we have come to better understand it as time has passed. While we will explore the discovery of deeper meaning in our struggles in Chapter 10, how well we can discover such meaning will be directly related to our ability to effectively work with the stress that comes as a byproduct of our loved one's illness. In examining how our thinking patterns impact stress, there is a risk that cognitively based strategies can be misinterpreted as an attempt to devalue the feelings, pain, and significance of our struggles—but that is not the case. Instead, the tools that follow are designed to help us accept, validate, and manage our emotions instead of fearing, suppressing, or avoiding them. Realizing this, let's explore coping tools for our mind with a focus on mastering care partner stress as experienced in the day-to-day interactions with our loved ones.

### Realistic Thinking

Thinking realistically is vital to our mental health. Realistic thinking is best summed up as having thoughts that are logical, true, and help us to manage stress while moving toward our goals. Unrealistic thinking is just the opposite: thinking that is illogical, inaccurate, and hurtful to our ability to manage stress and reach our goals. Whereas unrealistic thinking triggers fight-or-flight and leads to unhealthy stress responses, realistic thinking leads to reduced fight-or-flight reactions and improved coping due to its more accurate and less emotional assessment of our experiences.

When Tom was at Hofstra University learning about cognitive behavioral interventions back in the early 1980s, the book *A Practitioner's Guide to Rational-Emotive Therapy*[2] laid out various categories of thinking that contribute to tangled emotions, which are still useful today. Three emotion-tangling thoughts relevant to caregiving are called *awfulizing*, *low-tolerance thinking*, and *self-worth rating*.

## Awfulizing

*Awfulizing*, also termed *catastrophizing*, refers to the tendency to lose perspective on daily experiences. Awfulized thoughts can sound like:

- *This is awful* (or horrible, terrible, a disaster, etc.).
- *This is driving me crazy.*
- *This is overwhelming.*

While thoughts or statements like these are part of our common vocabulary, they can unintentionally lead to increased stress. Our brains tend to be very "audiovisual," which means that we will quickly visualize pictures of the words that we think or say. As an example, imagine that you are sitting in a quiet room looking at social media while a friend is in another room watching TV. Suddenly, that friend bursts in and yells, "Quick, come look at this disaster on TV!" What do you immediately picture you'll see on the television when you get to the other room? Most of us will picture some type of death and destruction scenario, like a bad accident, fire, tornado, etc. We don't sit back, yawn, and say to ourselves, *Gee, I wonder what this friend of mine might mean by the word* disaster . . . *Let me ponder this.* Instead, we jump up quickly to see what's on the TV and immediately feel a burst of tension. This connection between the words we hear and the pictures that pop into our head is automatic, and words like *awful, overwhelming,* and *terrible* easily create scary images that trigger fight-or-flight reactions, leading to increased heart rates, muscle tension, and even a sense of doom.

Early on, it was common for us to awfulize day-to-day experiences with Mom.

| MOM WOULD: | WE WOULD THINK/SAY TO OURSELVES: |
|---|---|
| Repeat the same thing over and over. | *Oh my God, this is ridiculous.* |
| Perseverate on a hallucination that children were in her room. | *This is bizarre.* |
| Accuse us of not caring about her. | *Holy \*\*\*\*. This is overwhelming.* |
| Call five or six times in a day. | *This is a nightmare.* |

Experiencing such symptoms of Mom's dementia was stressful enough, but, unknowingly, we were throwing gas on the stress fire by labeling those moments as *ridiculous, bizarre, a nightmare,* and *overwhelming.* Had we honestly asked ourselves, *Is thinking like this helping me manage my stress?*, the answer would have clearly been *no.* Those overgeneralized labels were stoking intensive fight-or-flight responses and were hurting our ability to manage stress, which made it harder to live our care partner goals like staying calm and patient.

Second, if we had paused to ask *Is what I'm thinking true?* we would have been able to see that, in those moments of Mom's repeating, perseverating, accusing, and making multiple phone calls, we were not being overwhelmed. To be truly *overwhelmed* means to be annihilated or wiped out, but we managed to live through those moments and carry on. They weren't pleasant moments, but we made it through. Also, what was happening with Mom was not ridiculous or bizarre, since her behaviors were very predictable for people who experience dementia, and we were not in a nightmare because we were quite awake, dealing with very challenging behaviors.

The care partner goal is to purposefully step back from these awfulized moments and see that rather than *overwhelming*, *terrible*, or *unbelievable*, such experiences are realistically *difficult, challenging, sad, frustrating, scary,* etc. These more realistic labels serve to lower the intensity of fight-or-flight responses, as they help you shift your appraisal of the experience from emotional danger to emotional discomfort. A helpful de-awfulizing tool is to create a coping vocabulary that allows for labeling difficult care partner moments with words that can reduce stress. While it is important to create your own vocabulary, here are some of the thought/phrases that we've found tremendously helpful:

## This is really _ _ _ _ _ _ _ _

| uncomfortable | disappointing | annoying |
|---|---|---|
| frustrating | heavy | challenging |
| difficult | troublesome | disconcerting |
| upsetting | sad | tough |

But how do you come to actually believe that these words and labels are true compared to the awfulized terms? Putting softer-sounding words in your head might sound nice, but they don't help anything unless you know that they are true. A phrase from John 8:32 in the Bible speaks to this—"The truth will set you free"—but those words are only part of a longer phrase. The full phrase reads: " . . . and you shall know the truth, and the truth will set you free." In other words, unless you know or fully understand the truth and reality of something, you remain trapped, and in this case, you remain emotionally trapped in stress. Then how can you know the truth of a de-awfulized perspective in care partnering? One way is to recognize that your own coping track record is being hidden by the next category of unrealistic thoughts.

## Low-Tolerance Thinking

Low-tolerance thoughts, or LTTs, refer to the ways we all unwittingly tell ourselves that we are incapable of coping with the stress that we're experiencing. Originally referred to as *low frustration tolerance thinking*, we can generalize the term to *low-tolerance thinking*, which can refer to any way that we imply we are unable to manage emotions and challenges. A close relative of awfulized thinking, low-tolerance statements translate into classic *I can't . . .* phrases that tangle their way into our care partner experiences:

- *I can't stand this anymore.*
- *I can't take it.*
- *I can't deal with another day of this.*
- *I can't handle this sadness.*

Other versions of low-tolerance statements can sound like:

- *This is killing me.*
- *I'm losing my mind.*

As with awfulizing, first ask yourself, "Is thinking like this helping me manage my stress?" The answer is no, since LTTs contribute to increased fight-or-flight responses. Thoughts like *I can't stand this* are tension-loaded phrases that send messages of threat and doom to your brain's survival center, leading to heightened physiological reactions.

Consider what is implied by the words *I can't stand this*. The first two words, *I can't,* speak to powerlessness. If you were told that the secret to overcoming all care partner stress was to flap your arms like a bird and fly around the room for five minutes, what would you say? You would say, "I can't fly by flapping my arms." You would be right, since that is impossible . . . You are powerless to fly by flapping your arms, and your brain knows it. *I can't* means impossible.

What do the next words, *stand this,* literally mean? In a coping context, they technically translate as *survive this.* Without realizing it, when you say I *can't stand* an experience, you are telling your brain that you *can't survive* that experience. Since your brain's job is to make sure you survive threats and live, its only option is to shift to fight-or-flight mode, turn on the adrenaline pump, and rev up your heart rate, muscle tension, breathing speed, etc., all leading you to feel more stressed out and less able to cope.

As with awfulizing, the next question to ask yourself is, "Is thinking that I can't stand it *actually true? Is it realistic?"* Again, the answer is no. If *I can't stand this* means that *I can't survive this,* then given that you are alive to reflect on this very question, that's proof in itself that you did *survive.* The statement *I can't stand it* is false. If you're like us, you have probably used LTT statements thousands of times over the years and therefore have thousands of data points that prove *I can't stand it* is not accurate since you've survived every one of those experiences. The realistic perspective is that even though what you are dealing with in caring for your loved one is very difficult, you *will* deal with it. You may not like the way you are dealing with a situation in a given moment, but you can keep working to improve your coping in the next moment as you figure out how to deal more effectively with each challenge.

If a low-tolerance thought like *I can't stand it* is false, then what is true? Truth is found in realistic statements such as:

- *I can deal with this.*

- *I can cope with what's in front of me.*
- *I can handle this even if it's hard.*
- *I will work my way through it.*

As care partners, each day we get through validates the reality that we did survive that day's stress. Since we didn't die, each day validates that *discomfort* and *challenge* are the most realistic labels for our experiences. The most helpful, realistic, stress-managing perspective boils down to:

*What I'm experiencing is difficult and uncomfortable, but I can handle this.*

## Self-Worth Rating

Back in Chapter 6, we looked at how past experiences with loved ones contribute to developing core beliefs that can trigger stressful emotional reactions in care partner relationships. We established that just as dementia may intensify a person's difficult personality traits, dementia also has a way of intensifying difficult relationship dynamics between a care partner and a loved one. The resulting stress can activate a core of hurt that is echoed in personalized messages like:

- *I am bad.*
- *I'm incompetent and a failure.*
- *I'm weak and helpless.*
- *I am unlovable and unimportant.*

These thoughts surface when we are caught in an unrealistic thinking pattern called "self-worth rating."[3] Self-worth rating refers to the belief that the core of who we are as people can change depending on our experiences. On an individual level, for example, if I'm treated well, then I *am* good. If I'm treated poorly, then I *am* bad. If I do something good, then I *am* good. If I do something bad, then I *am* bad. These beliefs reflect a major external locus of control; not only are emotions controlled by experiences, but the actual essence of one's identity as a person is also defined by what happens. While operating under this assumption, it's very hard to avoid care partner stress, where anger, anxiety, sadness, and guilt can quickly spike.

Remember the example when Mom was critical of Donna and said that Donna never visited her when she had just done so the day before? Given Donna's childhood history of being in a caregiving role with Mom, the core message of "you're not good enough" led to Donna getting tangled in rip currents of guilt and frustration. Given how powerful the emotions flowing from these core themes can be, we will benefit from having a plan to guide us toward more realistic thinking regarding our personal identity, competence, and worth.

## Self-Acceptance

Realistic thinking regarding core psychological themes leads us toward healthy self-acceptance. We see self-acceptance as having a realistic appreciation for who we are as a person with an inherent essence of dignity, goodness, worth, and competence. This essence of dignity, goodness, worth, and competence exists at our core regardless of what happens to us in each moment or over a period of time. Sometimes it is hard to believe that such an unchanging essence can exist in today's world, driven by the perceived need for affirmation by others, material success, social media status, etc., but it does. Learning to recognize this reality of human essence requires understanding three things:

1. The difference between self-worth and self-esteem.
2. How to recognize that one's identity as a person is independent from our experiences.

3. How to prove that one's essence of dignity and worth endures beyond potentially invalidating and stressful care partner experiences.

## Self-Worth vs. Self-Esteem

Over the last several decades, *self-worth* and *self-esteem* have somehow become synonyms for each other. The terms get lumped together with other "self"-related words, like *self-image* or *self-concept*, understandably producing confusion. Such confusion contributes to care partner stress, as it leads to an increased tendency to personalize experiences with a loved one and worsens feelings like guilt and anger. To build a healthy self-acceptance, let's examine the distinction between self-worth and self-esteem.

### Self-Worth

*Self-worth* refers to someone's essence of goodness, competence, and dignity as a human person. This is an abstract concept, so let's break down the words *essence*, *goodness*, *competence*, and *dignity* into as concrete terms as possible.

*Essence*: A basic quality to being human. An essence quality is fundamental to our identity as a person. We are created with it as part of our very being. An essence quality is not a quality that is given to someone by another person; it is part of the fabric of who we are and can never be removed or lost. Self-worth as an essence quality means that it is present in us 100 percent of the time regardless of what we do, what we think of ourselves, or what others think about us.

*Goodness*: Goodness refers to someone's inherent capacity for having a positive or beneficial impact on the people or world around us. Even though we can all behave in ways that have negative impact, we never remove the capacity for the positive. Certainly, this concept leads to all kinds of interesting philosophical debates about human nature and what it means to be a person—though that's best left for another discussion. Our focus here is on who we are as people engaged in a care partner relationship and on the personhood of our loved one with dementia.

*Competence*: Similar to goodness, competence refers to the inherent capacity to successfully perform a task. We all have different competencies or levels of competency in doing a certain thing, but each of us possesses some ability to function in ways that maintain or enrich ourselves, other people, or our environment.

*Dignity*: Dignity is the concept that best sums up the essence of personal identity. Dignity is the intrinsic worth that each of us possesses. This worth deserves to be respected regardless of personal genetics, history, behavior, self-understanding, or situation. Possessing dignity does not mean that a given behavior must be approved; rather, the concept of dignity is an unalienable property of each person that transcends behavior, personality, and place in life. It also transcends suffering with dementia.

This essence of dignity implies two very important realities:

1. A person's essence of dignity is constantly present. It cannot change or vary. It cannot go up or down or in and out like the tide. It is a part of us from the moment we begin life and does not fluctuate or disappear depending on whether I am able to be independent and active or whether I must depend on others for my care.

2. A person's essence of dignity cannot be measured. It is infinite. If we were given the task to go out in our neighborhood and measure the human worth and dignity of our neighbors, we couldn't do it. There is no measuring stick for quantifying human dignity because it is not a measurable quality.

To make the abstract concept of *self-worth* more concrete, let's violate this last point and pretend self-worth is measurable and picture that when you begin life, you have within you a ten-gallon tank of self-worth. You didn't have to earn this ten-gallon self-worth tank—it is part of your basic essence of identity. There is a measuring gauge on that tank with a needle pointing to FULL, just like the gas gauge in your car after filling up at the gas station. Your tank is as full as any other human person, because all human beings have the same ten gallons of worth, hence you are as equally worthwhile and precious as anyone and share the same essence of dignity and capacity for goodness and competence. Now, every day afterward, since you remain an individual human being, you still have your inherent ten gallons of worth. The needle on the tank should still be pointing to full.

Here's the dilemma for most of us: While our self-worth tank needle should always point to full, we don't usually see it that way. Under the stress of caring for loved ones, a self-worth tank needle bounces from full to empty to half full and then back again, sometimes over the course of a day. But how can this happen if self-worth is supposed to be constant, unchanging, and basic to our identities? The fluctuations happen because of self-esteem.

## Self-Esteem

While *self-worth* refers to the essence of someone's identity as a person with human worth, *self-esteem* is totally different. Self-esteem is our *opinion* of our worth. Self-esteem isn't our unchanging, immeasurable essence; instead, it is a thought, an idea, or a judgment about how much worth, dignity, goodness, or competence we have at a given moment. How well we regard ourselves becomes hurtful when we turn that judgmental, critical process inward and begin to beat ourselves up, which, in turn, lowers our self-esteem.

We identified above that self-worth has two important essence properties: It can't be measured, and it can't change. Self-esteem, on the other hand, is different since, first, self-esteem implies measurement. The word *self-esteem* is rarely used without one or two small words in front of it. When you hear a phrase like "That person has ____ self-esteem," what word might you typically put in that blank? Most commonly, words like *low* or *high*, *good* or *bad*, or *positive* or *negative* are inserted. Words like these imply measurement, and in fact, self-esteem can be measured with various psychological tests that produce a self-esteem score. If we assume that my self-esteem is my self-worth, then we risk increasing stress by believing that our self-worth can also be measured and compared to others.

Second, self-esteem implies change. If our self-esteem is low, we assume that we need to find some way to make it higher. If self-esteem is already high, then we want it to stay there and not go lower. Both outlooks imply that self-esteem is variable; it is not a constant. If we assume that self-esteem is the same as self-worth, then we will believe that self-worth can change and thus reinforce the same stress that measurement of worth brings about.

In the context of the self-worth tank, believing that self-worth and self-esteem are the same fuels the fear that human worth is also changeable and measurable. This leads to believing that if your self-esteem is low then your worth must also be low, which is the process of self-worth rating in action. Such a process only invites more stress.

A good step in building more realistic self-esteem or self-acceptance is to consider ways that we already understand the differences between worth and esteem on other levels. Take money, for example. Let's say you're walking along the beach with a friend and you find a $100 bill floating in a tide pool. You pick it up and the following conversation takes place:

> You: "Uh-oh, somebody must have lost this. Let's turn it in and who knows, if no one claims it, then we can either buy dinner or donate it somewhere."

Your friend: "Stop it. Have you lost your mind? Money found in tide pools is worthless. It's wet, sandy, and has no value. It will never buy anything or help anyone in need. In fact, if you think this bill is worth even a penny, then you're completely clueless. Give it to me. (Taking it from you.) Now watch me. See, I'm crumpling it up and burying it in the sand."

What would you do? Odds are you would uncover the $100 bill, uncrumple it, try to find its owner, or keep it. Why? In context of our worth and esteem discussion, you would pick up the bill and do something productive with it because you are operating with a "realistic money-esteem." In other words, your money-esteem (your opinion of the worth of the bill) matches the actual worth of the bill ($100), which was given to it by the US Treasury. Your friend, however, is operating with "low money-esteem," which is an unrealistic and incorrect opinion of the bill's actual worth. You intuitively know that your friend's judgments about the money aren't accurate. Your realistic money-esteem is based on your lifetime of experience learning about the realities of money. In addition, this knowledge allows you to avoid taking your friend's comments personally. Even though you were called "clueless," you know that's not true and that your knowledge of money-worth (and your intelligence) is intact. You realize that your friend's comments are driven by low money-esteem and aren't a valid definition of you as a person in any way.

It would be wonderful if our life experiences taught us the same distinction between self-worth and self-esteem as they have about money-worth and money-esteem. Unfortunately, that isn't the case for most of us. By the time we've entered our care partner roles with our loved ones, we likely have had many difficult life experiences that blurred the difference between worth and esteem. Once blurred, it was easy to assume that inadequacy, vulnerability, or unimportance were part of our identity. Using the difference between self-worth and self-esteem now allows for recognition that the core of a person's identity is not defined by one's experiences.

## Identity Independence

We feel guilty when a decision we make with Mom leads us to question our competence as care partners and our goodness as daughter or son-in-law. Judgment and self-criticism of ourselves as bad, inadequate, weak, etc., is commonly triggered in situations such as:

- Not taking Mom out to a restaurant because we're worried she'd take forever to eat, get confused, or have to use the bathroom.
- Snapping at her out of frustration after answering the same question six times in twenty minutes.
- Forgetting to make a physician's appointment that she asked us to make.
- Realizing that Mom could no longer be cared for safely at home and beginning discussions about placement in an assisted-living facility.

Working our way through feelings of guilt, anger, sadness, etc., and growing in self-acceptance requires that we not personalize these kinds of care partner experiences and trust that we possess an identity independence. The example of the $100 bill in the tide pool showed that regardless of what your friend thought of the worth of the paper bill, it didn't change the reality that it was still a $100 bill. In other words, the bill had an identity independence, meaning it had an identity that was independent of how it was viewed and treated. To recognize our own identity independence, we can follow these steps:

1. Make a concrete description of yourself by filling out this Identity Independence tool.

### Who Am I?

NAME _____
STREET ADDRESS _____
TOWN OR CITY _____ STATE _____
COUNTRY _____
HAIR COLOR _____ EYE COLOR _____ HT. _____
MOTHER'S NAME _____ FATHER'S NAME _____
SIBLINGS' NAMES _____
INTERESTS/HOBBIES/ACTIVITIES: _____
HOMETOWN _____
NAME OF A CHILDHOOD FRIEND _____
ELEMENTARY SCHOOL _____
A PLACE I'VE VACATIONED _____

### 12 Personality Qualities That I Like about Myself:

(Do not use a "perfection standard" in identifying these qualities. If you demonstrate a quality just one time, you possess the capacity for this quality, so it belongs on your list.)

_____   _____   _____
_____   _____   _____
_____   _____   _____
_____   _____   _____

### One Thing I Like in Each of These Categories:

FOOD _____   BEVERAGE _____   COLOR _____
SPORT _____   HOLIDAY _____   SEASON _____
SONG _____   MUSICIAN _____   MOVIE _____

2. Realize that this description of yourself, even if only very brief and concrete, sets you apart from every other human being that has ever lived. There is no one else in the history of humanity that has your name, lives where you live, looks the way you look, has those family members, interests, experiences, preferences, etc. No one else has, nor has ever had, your specific combination of those identity details. This brief self-description shows that you are an individual human person and therefore possess an essence of dignity, goodness, competence, and worth.

3. Now think of a recent experience that resulted in your feeling down on yourself and experiencing a lower self-esteem. This can be an experience related to caring for your loved one or any other low self-esteem moment. Consider each step of this sequence:

   a. Right before this event occurred, you were the person described by this list. This is your identity.

   b. As the event occurred, thoughts and feelings were generated that led to experiencing low self-esteem and, figuratively, lowering the gauge on your self-worth tank.

   c. Answer this question: At the end of the event, with your self-esteem gauge reading lower, did any of the information on your Who Am I list change? The question is *not* whether you would you *add* anything to the list; the question is whether the event or the way you were feeling after it resulted in any of your identifying qualities being changed. Did your name, address, hair color, mother's name, hometown, personality trait, preferred food, etc., change?

   d. Realize that the answer to this question is no. Nothing on that list changed because of the event or because of how you were thinking and feeling. In other words, you have an identity that is independent of that experience. What happened has no power to define who you are as a person.

4. Now think of a recent experience that resulted in feeling good about yourself and experiencing a boost in self-esteem. This can be an experience related to caring for your loved one or any other higher self-esteem moment. Consider this sequence:

   a. Right before this more positive event occurred, you were the person described by this list. This is your identity.

   b. As this event occurred, thoughts and feelings were generated that led to experiencing raised self-esteem, and, figuratively, raising the gauge on your self-worth tank.

   c. Answer this question: At the end of the event, with your self-esteem gauge reading higher, did any of the information on your Who Am I list change? The question is *not* whether you would you *add* anything to the list; the question is whether the event or the way you were feeling after resulted in identifying qualities being changed. Did your name, eye color, father's name, or childhood friend change?

   d. Realize that the answer to this question is no. Nothing on that list changed because of the event or because of how you were thinking and feeling. In other words, you have an identity that is independent of that experience. What happened has no power to define who you are as a person.

The more you stop personalizing experiences and realize that you are a good, competent, worthwhile person independent from your difficult care partner challenges, the better you will be at coping with stress, especially because it becomes easier to separate experience from identity. Realistic perspectives are reflected in thoughts such as:

- *I may not have handled my feelings adequately, but I am not inadequate.*
- *I did that badly, but I am not bad.*
- *She may have said I'm stupid, but I am still the same competent person.*
- *I am feeling anxious and stressed, but I am not weak.*

Like the other tools we've identified, the skills of identity independence and self-acceptance take a lot of practice. We suggest you take a picture of your Who Am I list with your phone and keep it handy so that you can test out the identity independence principle every day. When an experience happens, whether it is pleasant or unpleasant, open the list and ask yourself, "Ok, this just happened, but has anything changed on my list?" The answer will be no, as nothing can change on that list unless you choose to change it (and some things you can never change). As you review this in your mind, reinforce these statements to yourself each time:

- *Who I am is not defined by what is happening.*
- *My identity is independent from this experience, and I am still the same good, competent, and worthwhile person.*

## Mindfulness

Realistic thinking as a coping strategy for stress can be quite powerful in helping you live a fuller self-acceptance. It helps you recognize that you can handle the discomforts that come as you care for your loved ones with dementia. There is one significant roadblock, however, to always thinking realistically: You are human! We humans do not think logically and realistically every moment of every day, so another important set of tools for coping that can facilitate stress reduction, especially when it is tough to think logically, is often referred to as *mindfulness*.[4]

Mindfulness refers to being aware of our internal and external experiences in each moment. You are being "mindful" when you:

1. Notice your thoughts, feelings, and body reactions.
2. Accept your thoughts, feelings, and body reactions without judging them in ways that take you out of the moment.
3. Choose how you want to respond to a situation in ways that we believe are important and best reflect your values.

To better understand this concept of mindfulness, consider this: As you've been reading, how much conscious time have you spent thinking about the sensation of your feet on the floor? Most likely you haven't been aware of it. Right now, however, you're probably noticing how your foot feels simply because your attention has been drawn to it. You may notice a small pressure on the sole or side of your foot. Interestingly, your brain was receiving that kind of sensory input, but you weren't consciously noticing it before now because your brain knew it wasn't important. You're noticing it more now, but you're not letting it stop you from reading and trying to make sense of the point of this paragraph. In other words, you're being *mindful* of the sensations in your feet. You're *noticing* the feeling and *accepting* that it's there but *choosing* to continue concentrating on your reading. This mindfulness concept can now be applied to mastering care partner stress.

As an example, Mom will sometimes call our house at 2 a.m. Being jolted out of a sound sleep can produce two very different reactions. On a given night, Tom's reaction is to spring up from bed and say something like, "Oh no, what now? This is crazy. Doesn't she get it's 2 a.m.? I can't take this." His heartbeat accelerates as he answers the phone, and his tone with Mom can be sharp and curt. Needless to say, it's hard to fall back to sleep after the call.

Donna's reaction might be quite different. When the phone wakes her up, her first response is to take a breath and register *OK, the phone is ringing, it's 2:00, it's Mom calling. It's not the facility calling, so it's probably not an emergency. I'm tense and frustrated with being woken up, but I can handle this. Now, do I want to answer the phone or let this one go?* If she answers the phone, she calmly asks, "Hi, Mom, what's up?" Whether she answers or not, she more easily falls back to sleep. In this example, Donna is adopting the mindful approach as she observes the experience and her reaction objectively, accepts the reality of it, and then chooses to handle the situation according to what she believes to be the best response.

Mental health professionals have shown that if we live the three skills of *noticing*, *accepting*, and *choosing*, then stress levels are lower.[5] When we incorrectly judge our experiences as threatening to emotional stability, as with awfulizing and low frustration, we are in a non-mindful mode, which triggers fight-or-flight responses. We all have decades of thinking habits that are hard to change. But with consistent practice, living mindfully is achievable, even when our best efforts to think logically fall short.

In Chapter 7, we looked at grounding tools such as calm breathing and sensory awareness strategies. These are useful as mindfulness practices as they help us to focus on the present. One way to translate sensory focus into a relaxing mindfulness exercise would be to:

1. Sit or lie down with your eyes closed.
2. Start to breathe slowly and calmly in and out through your nose.
3. Focus your attention on your nostrils and the sensation of the air moving in and out as you breathe.
4. Try to keep your attention focused only on the sensation at your nostrils. Whenever a distracting thought comes into mind, let it pass by without judging it, then return your attention to the sensation of your breathing at your nostrils.

Letting a thought pass without judging it involves what are sometimes called "defusion strategies,"[6] which we refer to as having a "NAC" for coping. Let's say you're practicing the above exercise during a lunch break at work. Out of the blue, you feel yourself tense up when you think *Did I call to schedule Dad's doctor appointment?* You'd be exercising a NAC for coping if you:

- **N**otice the thought. (*Oh, I'm thinking about whether I remembered to call Dad's physician.*)
- **A**ccept the thought. (*It's just a thought. I can just let it go and focus back on my breathing at my nostrils. I can deal with the appointment later.*)
- **C**hoose to refocus on my breathing (or other sensation) as the thought passes.

Practicing an exercise like this for fifteen to twenty minutes a day is a terrific stress reliever, especially in how it helps you prepare for stress triggers that occur during care partner activities. Let's say, for example, your loved one says that you never told her the time of today's physician appointment even though you told her several times and also wrote it down in her calendar. You start to feel a rise in frustration and anger, your shoulders tense up, and your lips purse as you get ready to snap back a reply. Shifting to NAC mode lets you respond as follows:

*OK, I'm starting to feel mad, I'm tensing up and thinking that she should know that I told her and that this is driving me crazy. Remember these are just thoughts; I don't have to engage in this battle, and I can just take a slow breath and start helping her get ready for the appointment.*

## A Picture Is Worth a Thousand Words

An additional tool in mindfully managing stress is using visual images or metaphors that can help our brain detach from fight-or-flight mode.

There are countless creative visual metaphors that help a stressful moment pass without judging it as a threat,[7] and an image that has worked well for us is a shark swimming in an aquarium.

Picture that you are standing outside of a large, circular fish tank at an aquarium. As you watch the fish swim around the tank, you notice many beautiful species with various colors and shapes. Suddenly, from the shadows in the back of the tank, you notice a large great white shark swimming toward you along the inside of the tank. Within seconds, the shark is in front of you and only an arm's length from your head. It is so close that it is blocking your view of everything else in the tank. Instead of running away or banging on the glass and yelling at the shark to move, you notice, in detail, the shark's body, its eyes, gills, teeth, fins, etc. You don't tell the shark that it shouldn't be there and that you can't stand that it's messing up your view of the other fish. Instead, you calmly watch as it swims by. As it moves away, you then turn your attention back to the other fish that you were enjoying before the shark arrived.

We love that image because it helps make a great point about stress reduction: If the experience of the aquarium was happening in real life, would you run away when the shark swam close to you? No, of course not. You'd stay because your brain knows there is thick protective glass between you and the shark and there is no real danger—hence no fight-or-flight response. That is what allows you to calmly let the shark pass, then return your focus to the other creatures in the tank.

Many aspects of caring for your loved one with dementia are like the shark in the aquarium tank. Stress triggers continually swim around in your care partner aquarium, sometimes dominating your thoughts and feelings in ways that seem to block out everything else in life. Rather than trying to push these sharks of stress away, if you can learn to notice their presence, accept the realities they bring, and then choose to let the tension pass by doing what you believe is important, you will reduce the intensity of your emotional reactions.

## WHATIFIO

One last coping tool for the mind targets the anxiety and stress related to the uncertainties involved in caring for someone with dementia. As we mentioned at the start, human brains hate uncertainty and when it's present will produce stress reactions in order to prepare for survival. Two of the most stress-intensifying words in caregiving are *what if*.

What if Mom falls and breaks her hip?

What if we haven't taken all the legal steps we need to take?

What if we run out of money?

What if these hallucinations never stop?

Each of us could produce a long list of *what ifs* that loom like very large, teeth-baring sharks of uncertainty. The quickest way we've found to help these sharks pass by is to use an exercise that pulls together many of the realistic thinking and mindfulness principles we've identified so far. It goes like this:

1. Take the words WHAT IF and write them vertically.

    W
    H
    A
    T
    I
    F

2. Then add the letters I and O at the end.

    W
    H
    A
    T
    I
    F
    I
    O

3. Each letter then stands for a word in the following coping statement:

**W**hatever
**H**appens
**A**bout
**T**his
**I**'ll
**F**igure
**I**t
**O**ut

"Whatever Happens About This, I'll Figure It Out" provides your brain with an antidote for uncertainty because it is true: Whatever happens as you care for your loved one in each day-to-day situation *will* get figured out in one way or another. You can trust that the calmer we remain as whatever occurs, the more effectively you'll figure out and deal with the challenge at hand. When we personally use WHATIFIO in action, we try to breath in slowly as we say to ourselves, "Whatever happens about this," and then breathe out slowly as we say, "I'll figure it out." When we believe in the truth of these eight words, our sharks will tend to swim away more quickly, and may even start to appear smaller and less threatening.

## Minding Our Minds

At the start of this chapter, on coping tools for our minds, we said that mastering our emotions and stress within our care partner roles happens best if we can develop more realistic and helpful thinking styles and mindfully manage the stress we experience when we're not able to keep those thinking styles so realistic and helpful.

The strategies we've identified in learning these skills just begin to scratch the surface of the stress-management wisdom that is available to us as care partners. More detailed techniques for developing realistic thinking and mindfulness skills can be accessed through many resources. Stress-management classes at local clinics and hospitals, care partner workshops, and self-help books for managing emotions[8] are terrific sources of support and guidance, and we strongly encourage you to pursue them.

When it comes to the need for support and guidance, we have learned that it is much harder to find balance and master the emotions of being partners in care if we try to go it alone. Looking back, one of the most powerful turning points for us in working through the stress of caring for Mom was realizing that the only way we could truly follow a direction like "don't panic" was to "yell for help."

# CHAPTER 9

# Yell for Help: Social Domains of Coping

As care partners, none of us knows exactly what lies ahead as our loved one's dementia progresses. We don't know for sure what demands will be placed on us or how we will meet those demands. The stress of uncertainty will always be intensified if we feel alone and unsupported and, over time, can lead to patterns of anxiety or depression that further undermine our health.

Up to this point, we've focused on ways of managing stress that target the development of our own individual coping abilities. These *intrapersonal* skills focus on what we can do to manage stress in our own thoughts and actions. To survive in an actual rip current, however, we're also advised to reach out for assistance by yelling for help from lifeguards or other swimmers around us. This same principle applies in our roles as care partners since, to better maintain our health, an *interpersonal* source of coping support is necessary for solid stress mastery. "Yelling for help" from other knowledgeable care partners helps reduce the uncertainties that lie ahead regarding dementia-related expectations, behaviors, emotions, and outcomes.

## Why We Don't Yell for Help

As a reference point in understanding the reluctance many of us feel in asking for support, we remember an ongoing point of tension from early in our marriage. On long car trips to unfamiliar places, I (Tom) would be driving, and Donna would be navigating using a paper map (yes, in the old days before map apps). Occasionally, we would get lost, which would produce two different reactions: I would assume Donna messed up while reading the map and Donna, knowing she didn't mess up, would say these seven words: "Why don't we stop and ask directions?"

While Donna's question was quite reasonable, it never sat well with me because I illogically translated Donna's seven words into three words that sent shock waves to my self-esteem: *I am incompetent.* My response would usually be an agitated reply: "No, it must be around here somewhere. I can find it." While these are now comical memories, the stress we experienced in those moments was driven by my assumption that *if I can do it alone, I am competent, but if I have to ask for help, then I am weak and a loser.*

Many messages in our culture tell us that we ought to be independent and that if we are not equipped enough to go it alone, then we are failures. Believing that we should go it alone as a care partner is an extension of such messages that easily discourage asking for help. Taking on all care partner responsibility by ourselves invariably ends up in burnout from an unreasonable stress load.

Our personal experience of this burnout began in our first year of caring for Mom because we thought our professional backgrounds gave us everything we needed to succeed on our own. We figured Donna's work as a physical therapist/home health-care manager and Tom's as a psychologist meant that we had all the necessary knowledge, insight, and skills to guide Mom on her walk with dementia and manage whatever emotional challenges came along. After months of encountering many unexpected rip currents, we realized that we didn't have all the answers and needed to seek help. Since then, our yelling for help has been answered at different times by family members, friends, local dementia care experts, professional counselors, and a monthly care partner support group. We know that if we hadn't admitted we were lost and asked for directions, we would have remained alone, our stress levels would have stayed much higher, and we likely would not have found the right care combinations that Mom needed.

Yelling for help is an ongoing process that requires two general skills: self-acceptance in knowing that asking for help is not a reflection of weakness or inadequacy, and knowledge about the caregiver support services in your local area.

## Self-Acceptance: Asking for Help as a Strength, Not a Weakness

Appling skills for self-acceptance to seeking help is challenging due to underlying assumptions that inhibit asking for assistance. These often sound like:

- *If I ask for help, then I will look weak.*
- *If I can't take care of him/her by myself, then I am a failure.*
- *If I have to rely on someone else, then I am inadequate.*
- *If I can't keep my promise to care for my loved one by myself, then I am bad.*

Assumptions like these are rooted in self-worth rating and the belief that our identity, competence, or worth can be defined by our experiences. If we believe that we must care for our loved one independently and that we are bad, weak, or a failure if we don't, we will quickly find ourselves floundering in a fast-moving rip current of emotions like guilt and frustration.

Acknowledging that you can't do it all alone and asking for advice benefits both yourself *and* your loved one, as dementia care guidance and emotional support can help reduce uncertainty. Allowing yourself to turn to others for help starts by applying the self-acceptance strategies for recognizing identity independence and realizing that asking for support does not reflect inadequacy.

To better understand these concepts, you can adapt the Identity Independence tool that you used in Chapter 8 to asking for support. Although it will seem familiar, the questions below are specific to yell-for-help situations. Follow these steps:

1. Refer to your completed "Who Am I" sheet from Chapter 8. If you don't have it, make a concrete description of yourself by filling it out here.

### Who Am I?

NAME _____

STREET ADDRESS _____

TOWN OR CITY _____ STATE _____

COUNTRY _____

HAIR COLOR _____ EYE COLOR _____ HT. _____

MOTHER'S NAME _____ FATHER'S NAME _____

SIBLINGS' NAMES _____

INTERESTS/HOBBIES/ACTIVITIES: _____

HOMETOWN _____

NAME OF A CHILDHOOD FRIEND _____

ELEMENTARY SCHOOL _____

A PLACE I'VE VACATIONED _____

## 12 Personality Qualities That I Like about Myself:

(Do not use a "perfection standard" in identifying these qualities. If you demonstrate a quality just one time, you possess the capacity for this quality, so it belongs on your list.)

_____    _____    _____
_____    _____    _____
_____    _____    _____
_____    _____    _____

## One Thing I Like in Each of These Categories:

FOOD _____    BEVERAGE _____    COLOR _____
SPORT _____    HOLIDAY _____    SEASON _____
SONG _____    MUSICIAN _____    MOVIE _____

2. Realize that this description of yourself, even if very brief and concrete, sets you apart from every other human being that has ever lived. There is no one else in the history of humanity that has your name, lives where you live, looks the way you look, has those family members, interests, experiences, preferences, etc. No one else has, nor has ever had, your specific combination of those identity details. This brief self-description shows that you are an individual human person with an essence of dignity, goodness, competence, and worth.

3. Picture yourself asking for and/or receiving help in caring for your loved one.

4. Consider this sequence:

    a. Right before asking for/receiving help, you are the person described by this list. This is your identity as a good, competent, worthwhile person.

b. Answer this question: After asking for/receiving help, did any of the information on your Who Am I list change? Did asking for/receiving help, or the way you are feeling about it, result in qualities being changed? Did your name, address, hair color, mother's name, hometown, etc., change?

c. Realize that the answer to this question is no. Nothing on that list changes because you asked for or received help. In other words, you have an identity that is independent from seeking support. Seeking help has no power to define or diminish who you are—meaning that even though you are seeking care partner help, you are still the same, good, competent person.

Hopefully, deepening this self-acceptance helps you see that seeking support doesn't mean you are selfish or weak. Seeking support is a personal strength that reflects an awareness of your limitations and allows you to begin adding an interpersonal dimension to managing care partner stress.

## The Caregiver Support Continuum

When being pulled away from shore in a rip current, a swimmer has a natural instinct to look back toward the beach. A swimmer knows where to find help and quickly scans for lifeguards or other sources of assistance. For caregivers of loved ones with dementia, knowing where to turn for help is not so instinctual.

In Chapter 4, we identified ways to find services for your loved one's care that ranged from physicians to home health care and day care services to assisted-living and skilled nursing facilities. Luckily, there is also a continuum of services that exists to support your own self-care.

## Family Members

All care partners hope that family members will be sources of empathy, understanding, and support during our care partner years. Having trusted relatives that share in the care partner process is a true blessing, and we feel that blessing whenever one of our family members can visit Mom or checks in by phone. In some families, the dynamics are more difficult, so it is important to talk together as a family about expectations for each other regarding care partner roles and responsibilities. Discussions that maintain open communication will be needed as family circumstances and a loved one's needs change over time. Often one family member takes primary responsibility for a loved one's care after an initial diagnosis of dementia. Since it is common that people with dementia need less care in the early stages of their illness, the initial care partner time demands—and stress levels—can be lower. As a loved one's difficulties increase, care partner time demands also increase, leading to higher stress levels. In successful family systems, when the initial care partner shares these developments and asks for more help, other family members respond empathetically and are able to create a plan to better share the care partner load. This can only occur when the initial caregiver raises the flag and asks for help.

As previously noted, patterns of family relationships are sometimes more difficult and do not allow for the trust and closeness that leads to mutual support in caring for a loved one. If this is your situation, it is still important to share care partner realities and challenges with family members, even via written communication if direct conversation is not possible. It's always best if such sharing remains respectful, honest, and focused on what is required to best meet your loved one's needs. If needed, setting up a family meeting with your loved one's physician or other health-care provider can provide an avenue for more objective discussions about care partner realities and options.

In the end, each individual care partner must identify the support desired from others on both a practical and emotional level. If those who you hope could provide what you desire can't provide it, you must figure out who can. There are many people beyond family circles who understand what the demands of caring for someone with dementia are like and can support you if you are open to asking for their help.

## Friends

Turning to friends for support will be another source of stress relief, especially when family members cannot be present due to geographical or emotional distance. Many of us often miss the opportunity for receiving the support of friends because we fear that asking for it will impose an unfair burden on our friendships. Even if friends offer unsolicited support, we often hesitate to accept it, fearing that doing so will result in our being judged as weak or bothersome. True friends, however, are always willing to provide support and don't judge us. Instead, our friendships deepen as we allow them into very difficult and very vulnerable parts of our lives. We have personally been touched by friends who have always been present, both in person and over the phone, through their listening, words of support, suggestions, and even visiting Mom and bringing her Communion on Sundays. Their presence has helped us feel less alone and motivated to maintain our friendships and spend meaningful time with those who care about us. Our friends have also enriched Mom's life by adding interaction into her gradually narrowing world.

If friends are not present to provide a shoulder to lean on—such as when you have recently relocated—networks of volunteers can be found through local churches or service organizations within your communities that offer to visit the ill or elderly. Regular or occasional visits by these volunteers can provide positive companionship to your loved ones, and these volunteers can become people to talk with as further sources of emotional support. In whatever ways it can happen, sharing your experiences and emotions of caregiving with others will always provide an important source of stress relief.

## Personal Physicians

Many of us only see our primary care physicians for annual checkups or for an occasional illness. Given the increasing awareness of the mind–body connection in the medical world, most visits to a physician's office these days will include some questions about the status of your emotional health. Hopefully, you will discuss care partner stress with your providers to get suggestions on how to effectively manage any evolving symptoms. Physicians can also be good sources for recommendations on other supportive services in the area to assist in your care partner plan. Remember, if you ignore or neglect your own health needs, you risk undermining your own well-being. If this happens, you risk undermining your own ability to care for your loved one in the best way possible. On an airplane, you are always instructed to put on your own oxygen mask before assisting someone else.

## Care Partner Support Agencies

We have referenced several groups that offer resources for obtaining care, such as the Alzheimer's Association, the National Association for Home Care and Hospice, etc. These and similar agencies can also be excellent resources for your own self-care. These resources can be found in print and on agency websites, but we are strong advocates for seeking out people you can talk to. There is power in human connections, which can be accessed by phone, in person, and online. We urge you to access such connections in whatever form best serves your needs. Contact information for the aforementioned resources, as well as many more, can be found in the Appendix.

## Phone Hotlines

Several national agencies offer caregiving support that is, literally, just a phone call away. Hotlines can connect us to trained support staff who can talk us through even the most difficult care partner situations at any time of day or night. We have known people who used hotlines following a series of stressful events with a loved one that had left them feeling very alone and fearful. Those conversations helped with anxiety, loneliness, problem-solving, and finding additional care partner resources. Contact information for hotlines offered by the Alzheimer's Association and the Alzheimer's Foundation of America can also be found in the Appendix.

## Educational Programs and Publications

Information about dementia is offered by many groups and professional associations. Publications are usually written in concise, easy-to-read formats that focus on key areas of concern such as the signs of dementia, legal issues, resources for care and support, etc. These publications can be read online, downloaded, or received by mail.

Educational programs range from short one-session seminars to multiple-session care partner training courses. Many programs are offered in person on a local basis, and most programs also have an online version as well. An advantage to the in-person formats is how they can lead to forming ongoing supportive relationships with other care partners and support professionals. You can search for publications and local programs through the organizations listed in the Appendix.

In addition to these national organizations, many local hospitals and health-care agencies offer both online and in-person training and support. We are blessed in our area with an active state chapter of the Alzheimer's Association and a local organization called the Center for Healthy Aging, which is operated through a local health-care network. We have often turned to staff from the Center for Healthy Aging for navigating uncertainty, loneliness, and stress.

## Care Partner Support Groups and Forums

Perhaps the most helpful balancing and stress-managing component of our personal care partner journey was joining a support group. Our group is sponsored through the local Alzheimer's Association and meets monthly. While we had met in person prior to COVID-19 restrictions, we continue to meet virtually post-pandemic, as our current group members live far and wide. When we were new to the group, we entered with little knowledge about what the future would hold. We also had some ambivalence about what the group would expect from us. From the beginning, however, we received reassurance from our group leader (a dementia specialist) and from the group members who had been caring for loved ones for some time. They all freely shared their knowledge and experience in ways that taught us that there were varied solutions for care partner challenges. We were also reassured to see that others felt the same tangled emotions that we were feeling and that our own sharing was accepted without judgment. These monthly meetings always help us sort out emotions, as we can bring to the group our latest experiences and take away from the group new insights, understanding, and, most of all, hope. We encourage you to find a group that fits your schedule and allows for consistent attendance in order to take advantage of the supportive relationships that form over time.

As with educational programs, support groups for people caring for loved ones with dementia can be found through local health-care organizations, dementia care facilities, churches, or community groups in your area. Local support groups can be found by using the Alzheimer's Association's Support Group Locator. If you prefer an online community discussion and messaging forum for care partner support, they sponsor ALZCONNECTED. Both resources are listed in the Appendix.

## Mental Health Counseling Services

Another possible step in the care partner support continuum is speaking with a mental health professional. Accessing direct mental health support may be a difficult step if we are stuck in assumptions that speaking to a counselor reflects personal weakness or mental illness. As we've shared, asking for help is not a measure of personal weakness, and mental health professionals can be especially helpful in guiding us in managing our emotions more effectively. We have personally taken this step over the years and found it to be enormously productive, especially in helping us understand how our core self-esteem issues were tangled in old relationship patterns with loved ones. Untangling these patterns resulted in some of our biggest gains in managing stress.

Speaking with mental health professionals also helps develop specific strategies for coping with spikes in anger, anxiety, and sadness. Dealing with themes of grief and loss also become important goals as loved ones progress through the phases of their illnesses. Finding a psychiatrist, psychologist, clinical social worker, marriage and family therapist, licensed mental health counselor, etc., can be difficult due to location and increased demand for services. Asking for referrals from friends, family, or health-care teams is important. Finding a mental health professional who understands the course of dementia as an illness as well as care partner demands is an extra blessing. Most health insurance companies maintain a listing of the mental health professionals available within their network, so contacting your health insurance provider is another option for obtaining referrals.

## Help Is a Yell Away

Yelling for help when fighting rip currents of stress and uncertainty is a critical interpersonal step for mastering emotions. Asking for help is a strength, and getting support from others with knowledge and experience as care partners will always contribute to achieving balance. Without such assistance, we are left feeling like we are trying to tread water by clinging to a big beach ball of emotion and believing that we must keep the beach ball underwater to survive. As all beach balls do, however, the more we try to push it underwater, the more it pushes back toward the surface—and that is exactly what "submerged" emotions do. The more we push them down and try to avoid them, the more they find ways of pushing back up and making themselves visible through a vast array of physical and mental health difficulties. We hope you will allow those emotions to surface when they may and seek out effective support from the family, friends, support groups, professionals, etc., that respond. It is so good to know that we are not alone.

**CHAPTER 10**

# Keep Your Eyes on the Shore: Discovering Deeper Meaning in Our Care Partner Relationships

Until this chapter, we've targeted practical ways of coping with the emotional challenges that come with serving as a care partner. In this chapter, we'd like to explore how coping can be strengthened by exploring a deeper sense of meaning and purpose in our care partner roles.

As with other challenges, it is hard to search for meaning when we feel like we are fighting for survival against the stress and twists and turns that care partnering brings. If we were caught in a rip current and being pulled away from the beach, for example, none of us would be thinking about the rich beauty and gifts of the ocean. We would be thinking about how to avoid drowning. In the sea of care partner stress, we may be keeping our head above the water by not panicking and calling for help, but what do we do next in order to survive and thrive?

# The Shore of Human Dignity

Rip current survival instructions spell out the next step: Keep your eyes on the shore. In other words, stay focused on where you want to go, and don't let what's happening distract you from the place you want to be. If you lose sight of the shore, you can become disoriented and start swimming directly back into the current itself. Staying focused on the shore keeps you oriented toward your goal, which creates the opportunity for finding a safer route back to the beach. (We will discuss that "safer route" in the next chapter.)

As a care partner, keeping your eyes on the shore does not mean hyper-focusing on the struggles of your experience. Instead, keeping your eyes on shore means staying focused on your loved one as a person with dignity, regardless of how a disease is causing them to change. It means maintaining an awareness that in every interaction you have, there is an opportunity to reaffirm that your loved one is still worthy of the same unconditional love, care, compassion, and understanding that people without cognitive impairments deserve.

We don't use the word *dignity* here as reference to a person's behavior or appearance (e.g., *his behavior was dignified*) or when describing someone's social status (e.g., *they did not respect the dignity of her office*). Remember that human dignity is more substantial. It reflects an all-encompassing inherent right to be respected and honored as a human person, regardless of behavior, experience, appearance, or stage of dementia. Dignity reflects the right to be loved and understood regardless of whether one's behavior is loving or understanding in return. Dignity is not earned; it is simply present within each of us.

Keeping your eyes on the dignity of your loved one allows you to look beneath dementia symptoms and see that your loved one's personhood remains and is still worthy of love, honor, and respect. It also means realizing that your care partner efforts and actions are the most important sources of dignity validation that your loved one can experience.

We believe that no matter how severe symptoms and the condition may have become, our loved ones still perceive that we love and value them. If care partnering is a song we sing, we trust that they will always sense a melody of love in our relationships, even when they are unable to understand the lyrics. Recognizing that we are a gift to our loved ones through this power to validate their dignity is not only deeply meaningful but also a stress-management reality. We cope more effectively with *any* difficulty when we find personal meaning within the struggle. As Pope John Paul II once wrote: " . . . the more we move about in the dark and unknown areas of human reality, the better we understand that it is in the more difficult and disturbing situations that the dignity and grandeur of the human being emerges."[1] This resonates true when caring for someone with dementia.

As much as we'd like to always keep our eyes focused on such meaning, we are imperfect people. Recently, Mom was again struggling with hallucinations of children in her room and delusions that someone wanted to buy one of her great-grandchildren. She was also increasingly having problems expressing herself and used many unintelligible nonsense words (sometimes called "word salad"). When things like this happen, it's easy for us to focus on our own frustrations and do things like changing the subject by pointing to the birds outside her window or showing her family pictures so we ourselves can feel more comfortable during the visit. When this happens, we lose sight of *her* and how we could first try to validate her own frustration in not being able to communicate clearly.

In moments like these, keeping our eyes on the shore of dignity means that we stop trying to swim against the current of her hallucinations and delusions and accept our own discomforts. Once we make that shift, it becomes easier to see that underneath Mom's symptoms, she is still a person who loves her family and is worried about the well-being of others. She is still the same person who has always needed reassurance to calm her fears and who deserves our gentleness in providing it. Sometimes, she will understand and be reassured by our statements like, "You still really care for those kids. That's such a good quality you have, and we'll go make sure that the kids are all OK." Other times, she is unable to process our reassurance and remains agitated with us. When that happens, we look for our next opportunity to offer a loving response that lets her know we're listening, that we love her, that we value her in our lives, and that we will make sure she is safe. We wish it was easier for us to stay patient and person-focused, but like Mom's own behavior, ours can also fluctuate.

## Shock and Impatience

From the introduction, you learned that a major reason we care partners have a hard time being patient is because our loved ones' dementia triggers a "disrupted equilibrium." The shock waves of this disruption rattle our nervous systems, stir up fight-or-flight reactions, and make it easy to lose sight of where we want to go. It's hard to feel and act lovingly when we're that stirred up.

There is an old, but powerful, short story by the American writer Nathaniel Hawthorne that captures how such a disrupted equilibrium makes us lose sight of the deeper dimensions of caring relationships. It's called "The Birth-Mark."[2] It is a story of a newly married couple, Georgiana and Aylmer. Georgiana was born with a birthmark on her cheek that she had always thought of as a "charm." Aylmer, a chemist of sorts, becomes stressed by it after they are married and decides he should try to remove the birthmark from her face. He says to Georgiana that her birthmark " . . . shocks me, as being the visible mark of earthly imperfection."

Through tears, Georgiana responds with what we think is one of the most profound statements of human nature in all of literature. She says, "Shocks you, my husband? Then why did you take me from my mother's side? *You cannot love what shocks you.*"

"You cannot love what shocks you." This is a psychological, emotional, and behavioral truth. If we are shocked by someone, then our brain has perceived that person as a threat to our well-being in some way. This shock is a tangle of fear, anger, or disgust that instinctively tells us to seek survival by fleeing in fear, fighting for control, or collapsing into helplessness. In Aylmer's case, he loses sight of how Georgiana feels about her "charm" and fights to control what shocks him by creating scientific concoctions to remove Georgiana's birthmark. In the end (spoiler alert), he succeeds in removing it; only the process poisons Georgiana, and she dies. Hawthorne's final words are a guide for us as we try to keep our eyes on the shore of our loved one. He says that Aylmer ". . . failed to look beyond the shadowy scope of time, and, living once for all in eternity, to find the perfect future in the present."

As care partners, it is difficult to "look beyond the shadowy scope of time" as we meet our loved ones' needs. We go through periods of stress and sadness when we don't see "the perfect future in the present," as we feel exhausted, worn out, and can do nothing more than cry in response to losing our loved ones a bit more each week. The stress we experience makes us judge what is happening to our loved ones as wrong and, just like Aylmer's judgment of Georgiana's birthmark, leads us to feel the shock to our equilibrium. This emotional jolt often results in a sense of unfairness.

## "It's Just Unfair"

Thinking about how unfair it is that a loved one has dementia, especially in its latter stages, seems to be another universal care partner experience. Unfairness can present itself in a single moment, like when a loved one is angry at us for no real reason, or it can present itself in the way we process long-term, heartbreaking grief.

It seems unjust that anyone should have to slowly lose their memories, mobility, awareness, etc., as they move toward their death. We have had periods of feeling exactly this way with Mom, over her eight years of living with dementia. To see her unable to recall the identities of family members is so sad and we often ask, "Why is this happening to her?" or "Why would God allow this?" It is very hard for us to search for and embrace a deeper meaning as care partners when we become stuck looking at the unfairness of it all.

Unfairness is like a shark near the shoreline. If I'm treading water in a rip current and trying to keep my eyes on shore but suddenly notice a large dorsal fin swimming next to me, all of my attention is certainly going to stay on that fin . . . and the large creature attached to it. There might be many wonderful people and places on the beach, but that's not where I put my attention. Watching that fin, I naturally assume it is attached to a shark that wants to eat me, and that assumption of vulnerability creates a panic that only further narrows my vision.

Luckily, the shark of unfairness is more like a whale shark. It may be the biggest shark in the ocean, but it is not dangerous, since it only eats zooplankton and not people. If I recognized the whale shark as a source of discomfort instead of danger, then my fight-or-flight reaction would be softened, and I'd have a much better chance of staying focused on the shore and surviving the rip current. Embracing and working through the discomfort of unfairness is necessary if we are to keep our eyes on our loved one, and we can benefit from another tool that can help get us there.

## "Should" Statements

In our discussion of building skills for internal locus of control and managing emotions, we identified three types of thoughts that increase emotional intensity: awfulizing, low-tolerance thinking, and self-worth rating. There is a fourth thinking component important in our experience of unfairness that is referred to as "should" statements.³ "Should" statements contribute to our perception that we are helpless in the face of unfairness and cloud our ability to see the deeper meaning in our care partner experience.

A "should" statement is an absolute rule placed onto an experience that is already violating that rule. (Be sure to read that several times, as it may sound confusing at first.) Let's say, for example, I get lost while driving (an experience). I think to myself, *I shouldn't have gotten lost!* (an absolute rule). That thought came to mind *after* I was already lost; therefore, my rule was already broken before I thought it. Typical care partner "should" statements sound like:

- "This just shouldn't be happening to us" (even though it's already happening to us).
- "You should remember what I told you!" (even though you already forgot).
- "I shouldn't feel so mad at him" (even though I'm already feeling mad at him).

"Should" statements come in many versions but all imply a situation-specific, absolute demand or law. "Should" statements can sound like "ought to," "need to," "have to," "got to," "must," or even certain ways we ask the question "Why?" For example, let's say I told my loved one the time of her upcoming dentist appointment. An hour later, she asks me the time of her dentist appointment. I could easily snap back with "*Why* don't you remember that? I just told you an hour ago!" Disguised in that "why" is the thought that she should have remembered what I told her. The rule *She should have remembered what I told her* entered my mind after she had already forgotten what I told her. In other words, my "should" statement rule was already broken before I thought it.

## Shifting "Shoulds"

Shifting "should" statements requires that we move our thinking away from absolute demands and toward thoughts that reflect desires and preferences. Preference thoughts recognize the true differences between a need and a desire. A *need* is something that leads directly to death if it is not fulfilled, like food, water, shelter, etc. A *desire* is a deeply held want or wish that leads to disappointment or difficulty if it isn't fulfilled. Unmet desires, however, do not lead directly to our demise. Consider the different emotional tones from these different thoughts:

| "SHOULD" STATEMENTS | PREFERENCE STATEMENTS |
| --- | --- |
| She should remember what I tell her. | I wish she'd remember what I tell her. |
| This shouldn't be happening to him. | I don't like what's happening to him. |
| There must be a way to stop her hallucinations. | It would be so helpful if someday there was a way to fix this; I hope that happens soon. |
| Why can't I stop getting so mad at him? | I'd like to stay calmer when I feel so upset. |

Emotional intensities of anger, sadness, guilt, and anxiety are lower when we think in preferences since they don't trigger loss-of-control fears and adrenaline bursts from our fight-or-flight system. In addition, preference thinking allows us to better access the realistic perspectives of the thinking categories we've previously identified.

| SELF-DEFEATING/HELPLESSNESS PERSPECTIVE | SELF-EMPOWERING/SELF-MASTERY PERSPECTIVE |
| --- | --- |
| This shouldn't be happening. | I wish this wasn't happening. |
| This is overwhelming. (Awfulizing) | This is really difficult for me today. |
| I can't stand this anymore. (Low tolerance) | I can handle this one day at a time. |
| I'm a bad son. (Self-worth rating) | I am still a good, worthwhile person. |

## Unfairness and Lack of Family Support

"Should" statements often appear related to family dynamics in which a sense of unequal responsibility is perceived or experienced. "Should" statements in these situations often sound like:

- They should spend more time with her.
- They need to understand how much stress this is putting on me.
- Why don't my siblings call once in a while?

"Should" statements like these can create growing resentment and spark angry conversations. One helpful perspective shift in this situation flows from understanding that it is difficult for family members who don't live locally or are less involved to fully understand the realities of a care partner process that they do not live on a day-to-day basis. Often, they are not on the front lines of decision-making, getting agitated phone calls, driving to medical appointments, etc., so they naturally don't register how hard these experiences are for frontline care partners. The "should"-driven anger we feel from unmet expectations for family members (i.e., "They should be different!") further drains our emotional energy. If we can move from "should" statements to preference statements such as, "I don't like that they don't understand, and I wish they could be more present," then we are in a better position to effectively manage our anger and hurt. We're also in a better position to find assertive and respectful ways to voice our concerns in hope that they may respond more supportively.

## Dimensions of Depth

The care partner "should" statement we find ourselves thinking most frequently is: *This shouldn't be happening to Mom; it's just not fair.* Through the lens of the heart, what Mom has gone through in living with dementia does seem unfair. Philosophically, it seems unjust, and she doesn't deserve any of the suffering and heartbreak that comes with her brain's slow deterioration.

Similarly, the heartbreak that any of us experience as care partners is also real, so we are not in any way implying that we shouldn't feel such heartbreak. Serving as a care partner brings heavy sadness, anger, and fear at many points in time. It is vital that we allow ourselves to embrace the reality of such emotion and express our grief and sadness. Doing so helps us better accept the reality that we are living. Yet, we also possess a capacity to move through the heaviness and keep growing in our ability to provide the love and support that loved ones need. In Helen Keller's words from her book *The Open Door*: "All the world is full of suffering . . . It is also full of overcoming."[4]

With preference thinking a part of our skill set for emotional coping, we are better equipped to keep our eyes on the shore of our loved one's dignity. As we do, there are other dimensions of meaning to be discovered that help support our own growth and emotional balance. The following five dimensions have been especially relevant for us.

## Transformation through Suffering

*Suffering* can be a frightening word. It triggers images of intractable pain, trauma, isolation, and being stripped of one's identity and dignity. Caring for someone with dementia, however, opens opportunities to see a bigger picture in which the experience of suffering leads to transformations that can improve lives and relationships. The word *suffering* has roots in the Latin word *sufferre*, to carry or to bear up under something that stresses or shocks us. We bear up under care partner stress with much greater resilience when we share our struggles with others. Doing so enables us to bear our pain in ways that allow for greater perseverance.

We personally experienced the transformative side of suffering through the way that caring for Mom has led us into a closer relationship with each other and with other care partners. We deal with stress more effectively, we've grown in our ability to be patient, and we are better at understanding who Mom is as a person. We've also grown in our relationship with her, as many past hurts have become less painful as we relate to who she is now and find new levels of healing and forgiveness.

Living the challenges of caregiving also brings opportunities to develop increased sensitivity to others who are living with dementia themselves or who are engaged as care partners. Bearing up under this stress develops empathy and intuitive awareness of what others need; we can appreciate their experience in ways that others can't. Perhaps this is like J.K. Rowling's Harry Potter, who is able to see the Thestral beasts at Hogwarts only after he has begun to find acceptance and meaning in the deaths of those close to him.[5] When we open ourselves to the pain and suffering that heartbreak brings and allow it to transform us, our acuity to see deeper meaning in each moment becomes sharpened.

## Simplicity in the Present

Learning to live in the present and value the simpler things in life is another dimension of meaning we discovered as care partners. Caring for Mom has been a gift in that it allows us opportunities to slow life down. Donna often says, "You can't rush dementia," meaning that when we are with Mom, we cannot make her go at our speed. Instead, we must go at her speed and slow down to the pace that she walks, talks, eats, or processes information. Every time we try to throttle up and make her go at our speed, she only becomes more agitated, and we only become more frustrated.

Slowing down and valuing the simple began for us during the earlier stages of Mom's illness as we noticed how much pleasure she was taking in "the little things." If we were out for a drive, for example, she would delight in seeing things that we never noticed. She would point out blooming flowers, different colors of houses along the road, creative door wreaths, etc. We once took her to a local orchard, figuring that its apple cider donuts would be the highlight of the outing. Instead, she was enthralled with the orchard's flowering apple trees and had us park at an overlook so she could delight in the beauty of the landscape. Another day, we took her to a park that was famous for its rose gardens. On that day, she could not remember ever seeing roses and did not know what to call them. Rather than be upset about it, she simply took delight in seeing them "for the first time" as she admired their colors, shapes, and delicateness.

Even in her own apartment, Mom teaches us to recognize the "perfect future in the present" when she responds with excitement and appreciation to common experiences like they are first-time events. She has had a small Gerbera daisy in her room for months, and every time it starts to sprout a new bud, she is filled with excitement about what is to come. Each time a finch lands on the bird feeder outside of her window, she lights up as if it is a long-lost friend. Each time we bring Mom her Friday night ice cream, she responds in gratitude with a huge smile, appreciating it as if she's never before had a mini-mint-brownie blizzard from Dairy Queen.

Yes, there are waves of sadness as we notice the changes in Mom, but she keeps showing us how to slow down and value the little things in our own experiences. We have become, for example, much better at sitting on our back deck and taking the time to appreciate the trees, flowers, and hummingbirds. We more deeply treasure time with our children, grandchildren, and friends. It still takes practice, but as we help each other bear the suffering that dementia brings, we strive to treasure the pleasure of simple moments and to remember that we can't rush dementia.

## A Gift to Others

As all of our loved ones lose familiar abilities and personality traits, it is natural that we grieve that loss, comparing them to the way they have always been. An unexpected dimension of meaning can be found in the way that they become a gift to others who only know our loved ones for the way they are today. Our sadness easily clouds our perception of how they often still make a difference in the lives of their friends, neighbors, and other care partners.

Throughout her time living in three different assisted-living situations, Mom has never lost her graciousness and sense of humor with those around her. Her current care partners tell us how much they enjoy Mom's ability to make them laugh with her spontaneous quips as she reacts to day-to-day experiences in the neighborhood. Mom instinctively expresses her gratitude to them for the care they provide, even during times when she is more agitated and struggling with her decreasing abilities. The staff often tells us how much of a difference Mom makes to them and how they love her personality and humor. At the same time, Mom looks out for neighbors on her floor. Over the years, she has helped them to eat meals, get to their rooms, and, most importantly, told them how good they are as people and how much she enjoys being with them.

When we are fixated on how much Mom has changed, we frame this as Mom being "less than" she was at an earlier time. Mom's care partners and neighbors, however, only know her for who she is now. They see her as whole and don't focus on Mom's missing parts because they've never known what's missing. This has helped us realize the value of not comparing Mom to the way she used to be. The more we move toward acceptance of Mom in her present being, the more we can appreciate who she is today and how she makes a difference to the people around her.

Doing so further helps us recognize how people with dementia make a difference to others on a broader scale. A friend of Donna's shared the experience of how her mother who had been living in a residential setting for people with dementia would often sing as she walked up and down the halls of the unit. Donna's friend said that she would feel embarrassed by her mother's behavior until, one day, a staff member told her how everyone on the floor viewed her mother as a source of tremendous joy. The residents and staff loved to hear her mother sing, and all felt that her mother was a gift to each person living and working there.

In Mom's case, one of her neighbors loved to paint small wooden figures, and painted one for Mom that she kept prominently displayed in her room. Mom felt very special that he took the time to do that for her. Whenever he passed by, she would always thank him and if we were present, she would have him come into her room so she could tell us in front of him how wonderful a person he is. He would leave with a wide smile and extra spunk in his step.

Another neighbor would often carry a stuffed animal with her. Even on Mom's most difficult days, whenever her neighbor would come by, Mom would immediately brighten up, smile, and talk with her about how beautiful the animal was and how happy Mom felt to have it for a visit. Mom's neighbor would be thrilled with such affirmation, which showed us, once again, that there is power in every moment to validate the dignity and significance of each person, regardless of their abilities. While we still can feel the pain of our loss, there is joy to be gained by valuing our loved ones in the present and trusting that they can still be a blessing to others.

## Deepening Love

At the start of this chapter, we discussed how our care partner efforts communicate love *to* our loved ones in ways that affirm their dignity and reassure them that they are neither alone nor forgotten. It is also meaningful to realize that through serving as their care partners, we can also deepen our love *for* our loved ones.

Staying focused on your loved one's dignity through acceptance, patience, and understanding creates an opportunity to know them in new ways. As Mom lived through the earlier stages of dementia, she experienced the common symptom of short-term memory decline. As is also common, her long-term memory remained intact for some time. As we spent time with her, conversations often turned to the past, and we heard stories of her youth, young adult, and early marriage years that we had never before heard. These stories gave us a window into what she was like back then and how life with her own family shaped her as a person. Her descriptions of the joys and pains of life with her parents gave us insight into why her personality developed as it did, and these insights helped us see some of Mom's behavior patterns in a different light. Other memories were quite humorous and provided glimpses into her past that were very humanizing, like when she and Donna's dad broke a bed while visiting friends or when she had to deal with an annoying neighbor who would constantly stand outside of her home and sing to the birds. Knowing all of this helped us appreciate Mom more deeply and led to an evolving acceptance, healing, and reconciliation that, in turn, opened us to a deepening of love for her.

## Witnessing to Love

One last dimension of discovering meaning is the way that caring for a loved one models a commitment to unconditional love and compassion. Love is sometimes understood only as a pleasant feeling that brings us joy and happiness. In our care partner roles, however, the difficult realities of sadness, anger, fear, and guilt are anything but joyful and happy. If we think that love is only a happy feeling, then it's easy to assume that when stress is present, love is absent. Keeping our eyes on the dignity of a loved one helps us understand that love isn't just a feeling; rather, it is also a choice to act in loving ways, even when we are not feeling joyful and happy.

Remaining committed to your care partner relationship even when struggle and strife are present serves as proof that love perseveres. Your caring helps instill hope in young and old alike that they, too, can love unconditionally and be unconditionally loved. As people observe your commitment to your loved one, it also reinforces that they possess human dignity that deserves affirmation and acceptance, regardless of suffering and struggle.

## Diving Deep

While keeping our eyes on the shore of a loved one's dignity and finding meaning in caregiving experiences is more philosophical than other strategies we've looked at for mastering stress, it is a powerful resource for improved coping and resiliency. The more meaning we discover in our struggles, the more effectively we will bear those struggles. Working through perceptions of unfairness that shock our systems, managing unrealistic "should" statements, and staying focused on the personhood of your loved one all help you bear suffering as an invitation to personal transformation. Learning to live more in the present, to value simple things in life, and to see a loved one as a gift to others all help us deepen our understanding of love and become models of love and hope for others.

Keeping your eyes on the shore also positions us for the final step of rip current/care partner survival: developing effective ways to interact and behave with your loved ones. So far we've explored:

- Preparing for the conditions we may face.
- Managing emotional reactions and not panicking when rip currents form.
- Yelling for help and support.
- Keeping your eyes on the shore of your loved one's dignity and personhood.

Now let's consider how to swim our way back to the beach.

## CHAPTER 11

# Swimming Sideways: Changing Our Care Partner Behavior

We briefly mentioned in the last chapter that keeping our eyes on the shore in a rip current helps us find a safe way back to the beach, but what exactly does that mean? How do we find such routes to safety? We know it's wrong to go with the instinct to swim straight toward the shore and into the rip current, since that will just tire us out. Instead, survival guidelines conclude with an instruction to act opposite to that instinct and swim sideways—that is, parallel—to the shore until we clear the rip current. Then, once we clear it, swim at an angle toward the beach using the incoming waves for assistance. Going opposite of our instincts is not only a physical lifesaver in a rip current but also an emotional lifesaver when facing the stress of a loved one's challenging behaviors, such as:

- Saying things that make no sense.

- Questioning the character of family and friends.
- Repeatedly asking the same questions.
- Criticizing us unfairly.
- Constantly losing important items.
- Insisting that something is true when it's false.

As an example, Mom will often confuse her sister, who lives in another state, with Donna. If Mom has a phone call with her sister, the next day she might meanly say to Donna, "Last night, why did you say that mean thing about our friend?" When this happens, Donna's first instinct is to feel a spike of anger and want to snap back at her "I didn't talk to you last night. What are you talking about?" At this stage in Mom's illness, however, responding that way is not going to help anybody so, instead, it's an opportunity for Donna to swim sideways and take a different route in the conversation.

> Mom: "Last night, why did you say that mean thing about our friend?"
> Donna: "Oh, what exactly did I say?"
> Mom: "I don't remember but you shouldn't have said it."
> Donna: "I don't remember either, but you sound upset about it."
> Mom: "I was."
> Donna: "What did you feel exactly?"
> Mom: "Worried that our friend might hear you say it and be mad."
> Donna: "So you felt worried about that."
> Mom: "Yes."
> Donna: "Well, next time I'll try to be better about what I say."

## Swimming Sideways: Changing Our Care Partner Behavior 135

Mom: "OK, that's good."
Donna: "It's a nice day outside, let's take a walk?"
Mom: "Yes."

In this conversation, Donna swam sideways when she resisted the instinct to correct Mom's description of what had happened and then connected to the worry that Mom was feeling. In doing so, Mom felt listened to, quickly calmed down, and we never heard anything else about the issue. Compare that to how the conversation might have gone had Donna given in to the instinct to correct Mom's perception and defend herself.

Mom: "Last night, why did you say that mean thing about our friend?"
Donna: "What are you talking about? I wasn't on the phone with you last night."
Mom: "Yes, you were!"
Donna: "No, I wasn't. I was at a show with Tom all evening."
Mom: "I know I talked to you."
Donna: "Maybe you talked to somebody else? Maybe you talked to your sister."
Mom: "You're my sister!"
Donna: "No, I'm not, I'm your daughter."
Mom: "You are my sister!"
Donna: "I'm your daughter, your second child."
Mom: "No, you're not!"

All the skills we've covered so far—preparation, managing emotions, seeking support, etc.—can guide our attempts to steer clear of interactions like this one and avoid being left in tangles of frustration and stress. Since swimming sideways is behavioral in nature, let's add a behavioral principle to our stress-management toolbox that can help us stay out of such care partner tensions: opposite action.

## Opposite Action

The concept of "opposite action" was first described in the early 1990s by Dr. Marsha Linehan.[1] In general, opposite action refers to recognizing when a feeling is not helpful to a situation and then doing the opposite of what that feeling "tells" us to do. If I am afraid to speak up in a meeting, for example, then making myself speak up would be acting opposite of that fear.

As we care for our loved ones, our emotional responses often lead us to correct them or change what they are doing. On a recent Mother's Day, our kids sent Mom two big bouquets of balloons. After a few weeks of balloons floating in her room, Mom seemed confused by the two bouquets and thought only one was hers. She wanted us to take one bunch away. At first, we pushed back on the idea, since we thought they were fun to have in the room. As Mom persisted and became more agitated, we eventually realized that we were the ones who wanted the celebration of Mother's Day to continue, while Mom's priority was the feeling of being overwhelmed with the size of the balloons. We wanted her to *fit into our reality* when, instead, what we needed to do was *enter her reality*. Donna was the first to recognize this. When she acted opposite of her initial instinct and agreed to take the balloons away, Mom settled down and was much happier.

Acting opposite of our instincts isn't always easy and frequently requires us to reach into our stress-management toolbox. Donna used some of those tools in the Mother's Day balloon situation. In the face of Mom's agitation, Donna was able to mindfully ground herself with calm breathing and shift to a coping framework in her thoughts:

*OK, this isn't what I wanted to happen. It's difficult now, but we can handle this and figure it out, so let's make a shift. What is it that* Mom *needs here?*

Swimming sideways (or opposite action) flows from the sum of knowing the conditions, not panicking, yelling for help, and keeping our eyes on the shore. Donna's handling of the balloon situation was a byproduct of many years of mastering stress through:

- Learning about the conditions of dementia.
- Learning not to panic and manage feelings through acceptance and realistic thinking.
- Seeking out and receiving support from many other caregivers and professionals.
- Keeping her eyes on Mom and the love they share.

Our goal, then, is to recognize when and how to apply the principle of opposite action in care partner situations while using stress-management tools. Over the years, we've lived by three principles, or proverbs, that have been extremely helpful in learning to let go of our expectations, act opposite of our initial instincts, and enter the reality of Mom's "moment." These three principles are:

1. Every time is the first time.
2. The only moment is this moment.
3. Listen, reassure, and change the subject.

# Principle 1: Every Time Is the First Time

A difficult part of our own care partner experience with Mom has been her declining memory. Mom's intelligence, recall of details, and ability to reason were always solid aspects of her personality, and while we may not have always agreed with her outlook on things, it was predictable and we always understood where she was coming from. As time has passed, however, she has lost clarity in her thinking processes, including loss of memory. Initially, her short-term memory deteriorated more quickly than her long-term memory, but she now struggles with long-term memory as well. This impacted our time together in many ways, especially as we lost the ability to share a continuity of life experiences that formed the narrative of our life together. While deeply sad, this was also very frustrating. Several years ago, for example, Tom may have told Mom he was leaving in two days for a trip. Later that day, if they were talking on the phone, the conversation would sound like this:

> Tom: "So, I'm almost packed for my trip."
> Mom: "What trip?"
> Tom: "Don't you remember? I told you before, I'm leaving in two days."
> Mom: "No, you didn't."
> Tom: "Sure I did. Remember, I said I was going to Rome."
> Mom: "No, I'm sorry, but you never told me that. I would have remembered something like that."
> Tom: "Mom, I'm sure I told you."
> Mom: "You must be mistaken."

By the time the conversation would end, both would be feeling quite frustrated, and Tom would hang up from the call completely confused and unsure what to do.

What eventually helped us understand Mom's declining memory was comparing memory to the game of darts. When we're younger and our brains are free of disease, memory works like a game of darts you'd find in your favorite Irish pub. The darts are sturdy, sharp, and capable of sticking deeply into a firm dartboard. The darts would stay there forever if we didn't purposely pull them out. Dementia, however, makes memory more like a fabric dartboard with Velcro-tipped darts. The board itself and the Velcro on the darts will deteriorate, making it harder for the dart to stick as the months and years progress. With pub darts, I can be mad at myself for a bad throw and work to improve my skills for making the darts stick more consistently. With deteriorated Velcro darts, no matter how mad I get, nor how hard I try, they sometimes just don't stick.

Dementia makes your loved one's memory like worn Velcro darts. The more time progresses, the less their memories stick in their brain cells. If we adopt the "every time is the first time" principle, it will help us act opposite of our instincts and accept that we just can't make our loved ones' memories remain in place.

We have always loved the idiom, typically attributed to Theodore Roosevelt, that trying to get certain people to change is like nailing currant jelly to a wall.[2] In modern terms, "You can't nail Jell-O to a wall." We love Jell-O in all its forms and always rely on it when we need a refreshing snack. Mom has even come to rely on it as an important way to stay hydrated. For all the goodness of Jell-O, we have never entertained the idea that it would make a good wall decoration. No matter how hard we may try to nail jiggly Jell-O above our mantel in the family room, it's not going to turn out very well.

Expecting that you can talk your loved one into recovering a memory is like trying to nail Jell-O to the wall. Trying to make memory return does not create new circuits in your loved one's brain that can hold a new memory or access an old one. The alternative is to accept that every time you interact with your loved one, it may be without a link to past experiences. Even though this will bring sadness and/or frustration, these emotions remain softer if you can accept that every time may be the first time. Doing so will help keep you more clearly focused on your loved ones' needs and work to make care partner interactions more positive for all. Here are some guidelines we all can follow for reducing stress by embracing the principle that every time is the first time.

## Avoid Stating the Obvious

When your loved one doesn't remember something that was said or done, try to avoid phrases such as:

- "I already told you that."
- "Don't you remember?"
- "How could you forget that?"

Comments and questions like these only point to how your loved one's memory is failing. If your loved one could remember, then they would remember. If they can't remember, it is due to disease progression, not a character flaw. Rather than stating the obvious, we can act opposite by patiently restating what we've already said and being ready to do so repeatedly.

## Enter the Time Machine

A typical pattern of memory loss for someone with dementia is to lose newer memories before older memories. Your loved one will usually remember things from years ago more clearly than things from days or hours ago. Mom would frequently have a much easier time with conversations that allowed her to reminisce about the earlier days of her life than she did talking about events from the preceding week. If loved ones are struggling with conversation, it helps to turn the discussion toward past life experiences since there is a better possibility that the pub darts of the past are still on the memory board. We've found it helpful to keep pictures, photo albums, and yearbooks around to jump-start such time machine journeys.

## Greet When Meet

The first time your loved one calls you by the wrong name or forgets how you are related is one of the most difficult moments as a care partner. Although this may not happen to everyone, it is helpful to develop a habit of naming ourselves at the start of an interaction. If a loved one calls on the phone, answering with "Oh hi, Dad. It's Sue" may help orient them for a more successful conversation. Saying "Hi, it's me" or just "Hey there" can unintentionally set a loved one up for confusion. As the stages of dementia progress, we may even add more details into our greeting like "Hi, Dad, it's Bill, your redheaded son." Announcing ourselves by name as we walk into a loved one's room can serve the same purpose, especially if we approach from the front so a visual association to our name can occur right away. Keeping eye contact as we talk also helps interactions keep a smoother flow.

Should it happen that a loved one forgets your name or who you are, you can slowly and gently try to reidentify yourself. If it happens, however, that your loved one can't register who you are, it is still possible that the emotional centers of his or her brain are registering the melody of your love for them as you connect in patient and supportive ways. Being unable to recall your name doesn't necessarily mean that your loved one has forgotten who you are. It's also possible that your loved one is as shocked as you are about forgetting your name, leading to even more confusion in the moment. With Mom, we try to trust that she knows us even if she can't name us.

## Principle 2: The Only Moment Is This Moment

Earlier we discussed the concept of mindfulness as a component of good stress mastery. As a quick review, mindfulness refers to:

- Noticing our thoughts, feelings, and reactions to our experiences.
- Accepting these thoughts, feelings, and reactions without judging them.
- Choosing to act in ways that reflect our values and what we believe to be important.

When we're being mindful, we are "in the moment." The principle of "the only moment is this moment," however, also includes recognizing how your loved one is functioning "in the moment" and then making decisions about how to best respond to their actions. Beyond memory issues, this principle focuses on their declining cognitive capacities and how this leads to their experience of reality becoming different from our own. In other words, when your loved one's thoughts and behavior do not make logical sense, you need a plan for acting opposite and handling such situations in ways that benefit all.

In our early caregiving years, we did not understand how dementia stops people from accurately processing their experiences. We know now that human brains are extremely complex organs consisting of many cells and structures laid out through several layers. The efficiency of thinking, use of language, verbal and nonverbal reasoning, emotions, instincts, and information storage (memory) requires these cells and structures to be healthy and well connected so that information can be accurately inputted and stored. In this healthy mode, our brain can figure out how to use all that data to help us productively and meaningfully react to our world. Dementia interferes with that information-processing system, leading to disruptions in thinking and behavior patterns.

How this disruption happens can be compared to the following math problem.

$1 + 1 + 1 + 1 + 1 = ?$

# Swimming Sideways: Changing Our Care Partner Behavior 143

The answer, of course, is 5. We come to that conclusion because we input all the presented information, store it, understand what the symbols mean, draw on past memory to compute how the symbols relate to each other, and then arrive at a logical conclusion. Unfortunately, dementia dramatically distorts that information-processing system, leading people with dementia to conclusions that may make sense to them but makes no sense to others.

As a figurative example, let's say that instead of the conversation about a trip, Mom and Tom were having a conversation about this same math problem: 1 + 1 + 1 + 1 + 1 = ?

> Tom: "So, Mom, what is the answer to this problem?"
> Mom: "3."
> Tom: "No, it's 5."
> Mom: "No, it isn't."
> Tom: "Sure it is, just read it."
> Mom: "I am reading it. The answer is 3."
> Tom: "Mom, I'm telling you it's 5."
> Mom: "You must be mistaken."

While Mom's answer of 3 makes no sense to Tom (or to us), it likely makes total sense to her because when she looks at the math problem she sees:

> 1 + 1 +         1 = ?     instead of
>
> 1 + 1 + 1 + 1 + 1 = ?

Clearly, to Mom, 1 + 1 + 1 = 3. Her perception of the information is simply different from Tom's because dementia-driven organic changes in her brain cells create what amounts to a hole in her information processing that, in the end, prevents her reality from matching his reality. She cannot believe that the answer is 5 because the information she is working with is vastly different from what is written.

Difficulty processing information has recently shown itself in Mom's use of the phone. One day, someone came to visit her and tried to call Donna to say hello. When Donna didn't answer the call, Mom assumed that meant that something terrible had happened to Donna and became very agitated. Even though the visitor and other care partners tried to reassure her that Donna was safe, Mom didn't calm down until Donna visited later that day. Mom can also call our house and when we are not home, the answering machine picks up the call. Mom can no longer distinguish between the voicemail message and actually talking to Tom and will begin speaking to the voicemail as if she is in conversation with him. Again, Mom's current information-processing abilities lead her to believe her perceptions are true, and if we try to bring her back to see that they are not, we only risk triggering more unpleasant emotion. No matter how big the nail, the Jell-O is not going to stay on the wall.

Untangling this kind of emotion from a disagreement on the answer to a math problem is one thing, but it is much more difficult when a loved one's moments of confusion become accusatory, fearful, or bizarre and may even include delusions or hallucinations. Following are some guidelines for weaving the principle that "the only moment is this moment" into your care partner strategies.

## Read the Room

It is challenging as care partners to meet our loved ones where they are cognitively, emotionally, and behaviorally on any given day or hour. You may not know your loved one's frame of mind as you enter the room, but your time together will be better if you recognize how your loved one is doing at the moment you arrive. Sometimes you can ask other care partners for updates before you interact, but since moods, behaviors, and mental clarity can change quickly, it is best to enter in without any expectations. Good strategies include:

- Beginning interactions with calm tones and energy levels that allow you to get a read on your loved one's mental state. Avoid starting out with levels of activity that may be unsettling to your loved one, who may have difficulty shifting gears from sitting quietly in thought or engrossed in a TV show. Slowly easing into interactions with quieter conversation allows you to decide how to best meet your loved one in that moment.

- Adapting styles of interaction to match your loved one's changing cognitive capabilities. In our case, Mom always enjoyed Tom's dry sense of humor, puns, and dad jokes (perhaps begrudgingly). Sadly, she recently has become more concrete in her language processing and no longer understands his humor. (It can actually increase her confusion.) In reading the room, Tom has decided to keep conversation at more concrete levels that she can more easily understand and process.

- Reducing any potential distractions that may make your loved one have difficulty focusing on your interactions. Common examples are:
  » Loud noises
  » Large groups
  » Bright lights
  » New or noxious odors
  » Tight clothing
  » Clothing tags

Sometimes distractions suddenly appear in the most unexpected ways. Occasionally, for example, Mom becomes uncomfortable with a family picture in her room that she believes isn't hers. Rather than try to make her understand that it is hers, we will often just ask her if she'd like us to take it home. If she says yes, then we take it. We might bring it back later, replace it with a new one, or leave the space empty, but any of these options can improve her comfort level.

It is also important to make decisions about how television will fit into your interactions. Many loved ones watch a good deal of TV and become used to having it on, even in the background. TV is often on when we get together with Mom, and whether we turn it off, lower the volume, or just watch it with her will depend on her state of mind. We try to be consistent in asking her which she would prefer, and when she says she'd like to keep watching a show, we go with it even though we'd prefer to be engaging in some other way. There was a period when Mom loved to watch golf with us on weekends. She seemed to enjoy recognizing familiar players and making comments when players missed shots that she thought were easy to make. Then, one day, she stopped wanting to watch any golf at all. Initially, Tom kept asking if she wanted the golf on since he's a fan, but then had to accept that her golf-watching phase had passed.

Finally, be conscious of anything that can distract you from your interaction with your loved one and make it harder to read the room. Focusing on unimportant chores while you are interacting and looking at your cell phone are two common examples of distractions. It's best to leave activities like these for the times when you do not need to keep your attention focused on your loved one.

## Connect More, Correct Less

Most of us love to be right. Being human, it's easy to want to correct people when we hear them say something we know to be incorrect. With dementia, your loved one will say or do things incorrectly and, while this will be less frequent during early stages of dementia, it will increase over time. Let your goal in these instances be to minor on *correction* and major on *connection*. This applies to forgetfulness, as we discussed above, but it also applies to misinterpretations, confusions, odd behaviors, and illogical statements.

As an example, while watching one of her great-granddaughters' wedding ceremony via a video feed, Mom kept confusing her son with the groom. Earlier, Mom insisted that photos of her son and grandson were not of her son and grandson. We each initially tried to correct Mom's perceptions but, since she kept getting more and more frustrated with each attempt, we stopped trying to correct her, went with her flow, and ended up having an enjoyable time simply talking about the goodness of family while looking at the pictures and watching the ceremony.

Since Mom has gotten new dentures, she will sometimes get small pieces of food stuck in her teeth. She has developed a pattern of picking these pieces out with her fingers and holding them up for us to see. Initially, we would *correct* her by telling her to stop and put the piece of food in a tissue. Each time we did so, she would get upset and agitated but soon repeat the food picking. We eventually realized that we were also just getting ourselves frustrated with our attempts to correct her. Rather than keep correcting, we opted for connecting and began to just hand her a tissue as we kept on talking. After she wiped her fingers with the tissue, we'd put it in the trash can and move on without any tension. At moments like these, calm breathing and recognizing that "OK, this is a little gross or embarrassing, but I can deal with this" helped us to better stay in the moment with her.

An acquaintance of ours had a similar situation with his mother. She had developed a habit of collecting small items around the house and placing them in a change purse. These items could be paper clips, candy wrappers, and even small pieces of paper she would find on the floor and then roll into a ball. When the son saw the rolled-up papers in the purse, he told her that she shouldn't be picking up garbage and that he'd put them in the trash for her. Immediately, his mother became angry, saying that the papers were treasures that she had to protect. Rather than keep trying to nail his Jell-O to the wall of his mother's reality, he put the papers back in the purse and praised her for being so wise. She quickly calmed down and then they had a nice meal together. Again, target connection over correction.

## Be Short, Slow, Simple, and Sweet

Many of the above "swimming sideways" examples involve verbal communication in some form. Most care partners find that the best interactions with loved ones are those in which we use these three communication strategies:

- Use fewer words.
- Keep statements and instructions simple and concrete, giving one step at a time.
- Maintain gentle and positive tones.

### Stay Short

Many of us recall the classic *I Love Lucy* episode called "Lucy and Ethel at the Chocolate Factory." In the classic scene from that episode, Lucy and Ethel are charged with handling pieces of chocolate candy moving down a conveyor belt. When there are only a few pieces of candy to deal with, they do fine and their stress is low. Mayhem ensues when the number of candies moves beyond what they can comfortably process.

Our loved ones sometimes experience our words in the same way: They do better processing fewer words, as too many unintentionally leads to information overload and misunderstanding as they struggle to input, store, and process normal conversational speed and volume. Compare these responses to a loved one's question such as "How are the kids?":

a. "The kids are generally doing well with where they are all at. They just started school and the new schedules are challenging, but they seem to like the schoolwork and the various teachers that they have."

b. "The kids are good. School is off to a good start."

In the first answer, both the increase in the number and length of words, as well as the injection of different topics in the same sentence, makes it hard for a loved one to fully comprehend what we have said. The second answer, however, has a minimal number of words, shorter word length, and limits each sentence to one topic. Staying short allows for the best chance of understanding our answer and, maybe, even remembering it.

## Stay Slow

Lucy and Ethel's other issue in candy processing was that the pieces of candy came at them too quickly. At first, the slow pace of the pieces on the belt allowed things to stay under control; when they came at a fast pace, there were too many to handle. The same is true when talking with loved ones. If we speak to them like we speak to our friends or others with normal information-processing skills, then they can't clearly perceive the content and meaning of our communications.

If you have ever tried to learn a foreign language, you can relate to the problem of quickly spoken words. You want to understand and interpret what is being said, but in the beginning of your language learning, the words seem to run together and you can't make sense of them. This can be the same experience for your loved one, so they will benefit if we speak to them slowly and clearly.

## Stay Simple

Speaking too quickly becomes even more troublesome for loved ones when the content and context is too complex. "Staying simple" refers to remaining concrete in the content of our communications and avoiding abstract concepts. Since the ability to process information waxes and wanes, the more concrete our topics, the better chance a loved one has at staying engaged in conversation. Lately, Mom has had greater success in talking about the birds at her feeder, a cooking show on TV, flowers, and the weather compared to talking about family members, past friends, or her faith. Suggestions for staying simple and concrete to make processing easier include:

- Keeping explanations or answers to questions as short as possible.
    - » Harder: "I can't make it Friday since I have to work late, and I have other errands to take care of."
    - » Easier: "I'll see you on Saturday."
- Giving instructions one step at a time.
    - » Harder: "The clothes go in the drawer, the shoes under the bed, and the coats in the closet."
    - » Easier: "Let's put the clothes in the drawer." After this is completed . . .

"Let's put the shoes under the bed." After this is completed . . . "Now let's put the coats in the closet."

- Offering either/or options instead of asking open-ended questions.
    - » Harder: "What would you like to drink?"
    - » Easier: "To drink, would you like water or iced tea?"

(An open-ended question like "Do you want something to drink?" will frequently lead to a flat-out "no.")

- Allowing time to respond to questions or directions.

While there is no general agreement about how long we should wait for a loved one to answer a question or respond to an instruction, we know it takes much longer for someone with dementia to process information. We have had experiences where it took Mom fifteen to twenty seconds to answer a specific question. Her delayed replies have often been important, and we would have missed the opportunity to understand her had we moved on too quickly. We wonder how many missed opportunities we had in the past due to losing patience and jumping in to offer a response or change the question.

### Stay Sweet

We've often discussed the importance of staying calm and positive in our interactions with loved ones, and it is no different in areas of communication. Loved ones will always best understand if we keep our tone calm, light, and affirming. Doing so requires good preparation for our interactions and well-practiced skills in the management of emotion and self-acceptance. It is very hard to stay sweet when personalizing a barb that a loved one has just sent our way.

Staying sweet also applies to body language, especially in instances where patience is growing thin. Maintaining eye contact and keeping body language relaxed and open helps communication to flow into better interactions.

## Creative Calming

The principle of "the only moment is this moment" often involves unusual and creative ways for entering into a loved one's reality. Several years ago, Mom experienced a phase in which hallucinations were very active. She perceived that children were in her room and that many had taken up residence in her bed. At one point, she refused to get into the bed and, from that point on, would only sleep in her recliner. With her care partner team, we went through many attempts to help Mom return to her bed, but all were unsuccessful, and she remained insistent that she would only sleep in the recliner. We were not comfortable with this arrangement, and trying to change her mind only led to her feeling great distress. Once we saw that the debate about where to sleep was more upsetting to her than the hallucinations, we decided to embrace her reality and stop challenging her decision. After we did this, Mom became relaxed and actually began to sleep better than she had in some time.

On another occasion, Mom phoned Tom and they had the following phone conversation:

> Mom: "Hello, who is this?"
> Tom: "It's Tom."
> Mom: "Who?"
> Tom: "Hi, Mom, It's Tom."
> Mom: "I'm calling Donna."
> Tom: "Well, this is Tom. You must have pressed the wrong button."
> Mom: "Where is Donna?"
> Tom: "She's at work."
> Mom: "But I'm calling Donna."
> Tom: "Well, this is Tom, and my phone rang, so I'm thinking you hit the Tom button on the phone that is next to the Donna button."
> Mom: "But where is Donna?"
> Tom: "Donna is at work, and I am at home. Did you have a question?"
> Mom: "Who are you?"

Tom: "I'm Tom, Donna's husband, with the red hair. I bring you ice cream on Fridays."

Mom:(becoming agitated): "No, who are *you?*"

Tom: "I'm Tom."

Mom: "I know Tom, and you are not Tom."

Tom: "Yes, I am Tom. We have ice cream together on Fridays, then other times, Donna and I visit and we go for walks in the courtyard and to the entrance to see all the new buildings."

Mom (angrily): "No, you are not Tom!"

Tom: "Oh, you know what? You are right, but I know Tom."

Mom: "But who is in trouble?"

Tom: "Oh, you sound like you're worried someone is in trouble, that must be scary for you."

Mom: "Where is Tom?"

Tom: "Well, I will try to find Tom, but I know that he is OK and so is Donna and everyone else in your family."

Mom: "He's OK, no trouble?"

Tom: "Right, he is OK and no trouble. Tom and Donna and everyone else are fine, and they are all happy."

Mom (now speaking calmly): "Are you sure?"

Tom: "Yes, absolutely sure, and I will go and find Tom."

Mom: "Ok, then that's good. I go now."

Tom: "OK. I know that Tom and Donna and everyone loves you."

Mom: "Well, I love them too. Goodbye."

Unlike the sleeping-in-the-recliner experience that played out over several months, this conversation played out over several minutes but still reflects the importance of entering into a loved one's reality, even if it requires unusual actions as care partners. Initially, Tom did not register how upset Mom became at his trying to convince her that she was wrong about his identity. When he finally acted opposite of his instinct to argue for accuracy, he could attempt to creatively calm Mom's agitation by telling her that she was right about his not being Tom. For whatever reason, she felt relieved by this shift, and Tom was able to clarify her concern and offer reassurance.

There are countless ways that we care partners engage in creatively calming, and as long as safety issues are not involved, the willingness to accompany loved ones by immersing ourselves in their reality will usually reduce tension, especially when our creative calming includes the next principle.

## Principle 3: Listen, Reassure, and Change the Subject

The third principle for entering the moment of a loved one's experience in a creatively calming way is summed up in this guideline: listen, reassure, and change the subject. While the importance of listening to, reassuring, and redirecting a loved one has been woven into most of the stress-management topics we have already discussed, this principle has been so important for us that we'd like to highlight it.

### Listen

To truly listen, we must be fully present to who or what we are experiencing. Listening to the full sounds of a babbling brook, for example, requires a choice to quiet ourselves and center our attention on the water as it moves over rocks and pebbles. As we do, we harken to the nuances of the brook and discover the complexities and rhythms that give the brook its identity.

In the same way, truly listening, or harkening, to your loved one allows you to recognize the nuances and complexities in moment-to-moment experiences. This kind of listening entails not just using your ears to register words, but also listening with your eyes, hands, arms, and, most of all, hearts. In this way, you can better understand the meaning of your loved one's experiences and better let go of your own agendas and expectations. When you do, the two of you meet in the fullness of who you are as people at that particular moment of your lives. In order to do this well, it means listening for your loved one's emotions.

Earlier, we distinguished between feelings and thoughts. *Feelings* refer to physical or emotional states and, hopefully, you spent some time creating an emotional vocabulary for communicating feelings of happiness, sadness, anger, or fear. While this is useful for our own growth in managing stress, it is also wonderfully useful in helping us explore and understand our loved one's emotions. In the above phone conversation, the tide turned when Tom stopped debating and listened for the feeling underneath Mom's words and said, "Oh, you sound like you're worried someone is in trouble, that must be scary for you."

## Reflecting Emotions

A statement like the one Tom said to reassure Mom allows us to become an emotional mirror for loved ones and reflect their feelings back to them. Emotional reflection is powerful in the way it communicates the message that "you are heard, you are seen, and you are understood. You are important to me, and I will help you feel safe." Regardless of our history with recognizing and communicating emotions, it is always good to practice the skill of emotional reflection. While there isn't anything wrong with using a lead-in phrase like "What I hear you saying is . . ." it isn't necessary to begin reflection that way. Other options for reflecting feelings can include:

- Observations: "You sound angry." "You look sad."

- Questions: "Are you feeling angry?" "Are you feeling sad?"
- Statements of concern: "I'm worried that you're mad at me." "I'm concerned you're feeling down."

In the end, regardless of the words we use to reflect a loved one's emotions, entering into those emotions lets them know that we value what they are feeling. This validation brings a greater sense of safety and security, which often leads to a growing sense of calm following such emotional connection. This is even more important when symptoms progress, as the emotional circuits of the brain can remain operative after other brain functions have deteriorated.

### Exploring Emotions

Once emotions are identified and reflected, we can explore those feelings together. Productive exploration requires that we receive what a loved one is feeling without judging or criticizing those feelings. It is very easy to unintentionally invalidate feelings with statements like:

- "Oh, don't be silly, there's nothing to be mad about."
- "Being sad will just make you more depressed, so let's look on the bright side."
- "It upsets me to see you so upset, so would you please stop."

These are actual sentences that we have used that simply weren't helpful, and we are grateful to members of our support group who were role models for us in using more productive statements and questions for exploring emotions, like:

- "That sounds really hard for you, I'd like to hear more about it."
- "What is that feeling like for you?"
- "What goes through your mind when you're feeling that way?"

- "What seems to bring that feeling on for you?"

Again, any way that we phrase our exploration of feelings is fine if we are harkening with our hearts and open to receiving whatever we may hear in reply.

Emotional exploration, as with reflection, takes practice. We can practice it with other family members, friends, coworkers, or even with television or movie characters as we watch them act in shows and films (don't expect the characters to reply, of course). As we do, we're also likely to notice improving abilities in listening for other important concerns that loved ones try to communicate. These can include preferences of different kinds or physical discomforts and pain. When we know what a loved one's concerns entail, we put ourselves in the best position to provide reassurance.

## Reassure

There are varied and often unpredictable reasons causing a loved one's distress. Some reasons are logical, like when a urinary tract infection is present or shoes no longer fit correctly. These types of issues are resolved through concrete problem-solving and usually result in improved comfort.

Other reasons for distress are not so concrete or logical, such as when a loved one unrealistically fears that they are going to be evicted from their place of residence or believes a relative has suddenly died. Providing gentle, focused, and, sometimes, creative reassurance is a direct route to increasing a loved one's perception of safety and security. Since emotional insecurity is a trigger for fight-or-flight reactions, reassurance can contribute to the calming of those adrenaline spikes and help a loved one restore some sense of equilibrium.

There are times when reassurance is straightforward and very specific, as in moments when a loved one is worried that a physician appointment was missed. We say, "Oh, you're worried you missed Dr. Smith's appointment. Well, look here on the calendar . . . See, the appointment isn't until tomorrow."

Other times reassurance is more complex, as in moments when a loved one is hallucinating that three groups of people in the bedroom are upset because a care partner only brought an ice cream treat for the loved one but didn't bring ice cream for everyone. Now the loved one wants the care partner to distribute candy to all who are present. Pretending to distribute candy to the imaginary people may appear illogical, but it is a meaningful tool in reducing the loved one's distress.

Recently, Mom has been worried that we are selling our house. We are not selling it, but she is convinced that it is on the market. Donna has been great at listening for the fear underneath Mom's delusion and has been able to lovingly reflect the fear and reassure Mom that she understands how scary that idea is for her. (If we were to sell the house, Mom fears that we might move closer to our kids in other states and leave her alone.) Since Donna has been Mom's main caregiving lifeline, the vulnerability and fear that this brings for Mom is very intense. Each time Mom brings this up, Donna:

- Receives it calmly.
- Breathes slowly and applies her own emotional coping tools.
- Understands that every time is the first time and that Mom doesn't recall discussing this yesterday.
- Accepts that the only moment is this moment and reflects Mom's feeling with a statement like "You're still feeling frightened that we might be selling our house."
- Reassures Mom that the house is not for sale: "Well, I know how worried you are about that, since Tom and I live close to you. The good news is that we love our house and aren't selling it. We love living in our town and close to you. We love our

deck and all the flowers and trees around it, and we love having our kids and grandkids come there for visits. So, we're sure we are not selling our house. Speaking of the grandkids, would you like to see some new pictures of them?"

Reassurance can also be provided in ways other than words, such as through gentle physical contact. In the fear-of-the-house-sale example, Donna will gently take Mom's hand in her hands as she talks with her. This adds a physical dimension of reassurance, which reaffirms their connection. Donna will also sit in front of Mom at her eye level so that she can maintain eye contact with Mom as they speak. As people age, the opportunities for physical contact become fewer as the amount of time spent with other people is reduced. Eye contact, hand-holding, hugs, or a gentle hand placed on one's shoulder or head send messages of warmth, concern, presence, and reassurance.

## Change the Subject

With listening engaged and reassurance provided, that last line of Donna's above response highlights the third leg of distress reduction: changing the subject. Changing the subject is not an invalidation of a loved one's feelings; rather, it is a loving strategy that flows from listening and providing reassurance. Changing the subject creates new focus points of attention that can provide a source of soothing for a loved one's distress. Learning to do this with a parent can be hard, as it can initially seem disrespectful, but the way it helps a loved one refocus on something more soothing is worth our initial discomfort.

Consider an example of your loved one saying that her deceased spouse is coming for a dinner date. She says this to a friend in a phone conversation and the friend responds, "Oh, come on now, no dead person is coming to take you to dinner." Your loved one has just hung up the phone and is crying as you enter the room. How might you respond? You could agree with the friend and try to force your loved one into your reality by explaining that the spouse is dead, but that might lead to further debate and agitation (or both!). Or might you take the creative "listen, reassure, change the subject" approach?

> Care partner: "What's wrong, you seem so upset?"
> Loved one: "Lucy is saying that your father is dead."
> CP: "Oh my. That must have been upsetting to hear. It's made you so sad."
> LO: "She's a terrible friend. I can't stand her."
> CP: "Even though she's one of your best friends, you're really mad at her."
> LO: "How could she say such a horrible thing?"
> CP: "I honestly don't know; it must be very confusing. Sometimes friends can say hurtful things even though they still love us. What were you talking about?"
> LO: "I told her that your father is coming tonight to take me to dinner."
> CP: "Wow, Dad's coming to dinner? That's amazing. You must feel very excited about that, am I right?"
> LO: "I'm so happy I could scream."
> CP: "That sounds wonderfully happy. You two were so in love. What do you think it will be like to have dinner together?"
> LO: "I don't know, but our dates were always fun."
> CP: "What kind of dates did you used to go on together?"
> LO: "Well, we'd go dancing, to the movies, or just for walks in the park."
> CP: "How did you two meet each other anyway?"
> LO: "Well, let me tell you . . ."

Many care partners find that more successful changes of subject are ones that follow reassurance with a related subject that taps into a loved one's long-term memories. Since short-term memories tend to fade more quickly, memories from younger years allow for more vivid recall, which lends itself to better conversation and connection to more pleasant emotions. While there is no magical solution for every stressful or agitated state, the template of listening for emotions, offering reassurance, and a redirection to new subjects always has potential for helping loved ones return to a calmer state of mind.

Changes of subject will come in all shapes and sizes, but the more the new topic is related to the original theme, the better chance that the subject shift will feel smooth. Shifts in topic that are too different from the original topic will often not have the same positive outcomes. In the above dialogue, for example, the care partner could have responded in this way:

> Care partner: "What's wrong, you seem so upset?"
> Loved one: "Lucy is saying that your father is dead."
> CP: "Oh my. That must have been upsetting to hear. It's made you so sad."
> LO: "She's a terrible friend. I can't stand her."
> CP: "Even though she's one of your best friends, you're really mad at her."
> LO: "How could she say such a horrible thing?"
> CP: "I honestly don't know; it must be very confusing. Sometimes friends can say hurtful things even though they still love us. What were you talking about?"
> LO: "I told her that your father is coming tonight to take me to dinner."
> CP: "I see. So did you do any fun activities today?"

Shifting topics from dinner with the deceased spouse to the day's activities can be a difficult track change for someone with dementia. In addition, such an abrupt switch does run the risk of invalidating or devaluing a loved one's emotions. Shifting topics in the original conversation from dinner with the deceased spouse to aspects of the couple's relationship over the years allows for validating the emotions underneath the thoughts about dinner together and even offers opportunities for processing feelings of grief. The key is finding associated or parallel topics to the initial subject to create a bridge that lets your loved one cross from agitation to a greater sense of comfort.

Here is a change-the-subject example where a shift of topic attempted to create such a bridge:

> LO: "Someone stole my ring."
> CP: "Who do you think took it?"
> LO: "The man who comes in during the night."
> CP: "That's not very nice of him. Where did you ever get that ring anyway?"
> LO: "Why can't I drive anymore?"
> CP: "Are you upset that you can't drive?"
> LO: "Yes, of course I am. I never get to go anywhere."
> CP: "Then that makes total sense that you are upset about not driving. Where did you like to drive?"
> LO: "To the bakery and the post office."
> CP: "What was your most favorite car that you ever owned when you were younger?"
> LO: "Oh, for sure it was our red Thunderbird."
> CP: "What places did you like to drive to back then?"

Again, there is never a guarantee that even the smoothest change of subjects will get us where we want to go, but if we remember that our first objectives are to listen and reassure, then we stand a good chance of successfully helping loved ones cross from a state of tension to one of validation and comfort.

## Sideways Is the Wise Way

Acting opposite of our instinct to bring a loved one into our reality may never feel natural, but one thing is for sure: The more we resist entering a loved one's reality, the more our mutual stress levels will become tangled in increasing tension. Just like swimming into a rip current, we will become exhausted unless we can teach ourselves to "swim sideways" and out of the tension.

When we build skills for coping with our emotions and practice stress management, we will be in a much better position to embrace our loved ones in their individual "moment" and swim sideways using the principles of:

Every time is the first time.

The only moment is this moment.

Listen, reassure, and change the subject.

CHAPTER 12

# Untangled but Knotted in Love

As we close this exploration of creating balance and mastering care partner stress, it is our sincere hope that you have discovered useful tools and perspectives that allow for a more peaceful and meaningful experience of caring for your loved one. Knowing that a more peaceful experience is still full of moments when caring for someone with dementia does not feel at all peaceful, we trust that the stress-mastery strategies contained in these chapters have helped you in preparing for and navigating through the challenges of living as a care partner.

Comparing the care of someone with dementia to surviving ocean rip currents hopefully has been helpful for planning and managing the medical, legal, financial, and emotional realities brought to light by this illness. Along with planning, we hope that you also find the coping guidelines for staying calm, accessing support, focusing on your loved ones' dignity, and effective interaction to be beneficial in building a productive stress-mastery mindset. Since we are true believers in the old farming expression "When you're green you grow, when you're ripe you rot,"[1] please consult the resources listed in the Appendix for continued learning. A wide range of valuable information related to dementia care exists and is always evolving, so we hope you will "stay green" and keep developing your care partner skills.

Personally, we try to remain green as we rely on these same planning and coping components in our ongoing walk as care partners with Mom. Looking back, we started writing this book nearly five years ago. Writing about our experiences has been a format for us to process our experiences with Mom on many levels. At times, our writing has been more of a personal reflection. At other times, it has been more instructional. Both versions have allowed us the opportunity to consider where we were at a given point in our own care partner journey. It has given us the chance to take stock of how we were being impacted by Mom *and* to take stock of how she was being impacted by us. It has been an honor to walk with her through these phases of her life, and we do feel blessed by the privilege of caring for her as she cares for us in her own way.

As we write this final chapter, Mom has recently entered hospice care. Her progressing dementia and concurrent medical issues seem to be making her days on this side of eternity more difficult for her. We previously noted how important it is to have good people as partners in Mom's care, and we relied heavily on them in moving toward the decision for hospice. Many of us incorrectly assume when people begin hospice care that this means their deaths are imminent, but this isn't always true. Mom is doing OK, and the hospice team can care for her in the same room at her assisted-living facility that she has lived in for the last four years. We know that she will be reassured by the increased presence of caring professionals and volunteers as she nears the end of her life. The support provided to us as family members through the hospice process will also be invaluable. While we do not know the number of weeks, months, or years that Mom will continue to be with us, we do trust that this step is right for this phase of her journey.

We were recently reflecting on our care partner experiences over the years when Donna visualized Mom as a nesting doll. Nesting dolls are typically carved out of wood and consist of a series of distinct figures, each one smaller than the first, and placed one inside the other. Donna said that, over the years, we have been losing Mom in phases like a nesting doll. Back in 2015, we saw her as a generally independent eighty-eight-year-old. Since then, she seems to have gone through phases in which different parts of her have separated to reveal a different version of herself. She is still Mom, but there are new details that need to be explored and understood for us to appreciate the distinct qualities of how she sees herself and her world. What makes the nesting doll image extra challenging is that we are never sure when we will be looking at the littlest doll. We don't know if the way we experience Mom today will be the final way we know and remember her or if a new way of knowing her will be revealed. What we do know is that embracing her within this uncertainty is sometimes still hard; at other times it is less so, but always, it is filled with meaning.

We often wonder how well we have lived our care partner relationship with Mom through her nesting doll phases. We ask ourselves if we've seen growth toward the three outcomes we proposed as the targets for our entire discussion. Have we seen:

1. Improved psychological well-being?
2. Greater emotional consistency in our relationships with Mom?
3. The discovery of a deeper meaning in our caregiving relationship?

Most often, our answer is "Yes, we can see some growth, but we sure need to keep working on it."

As in most endeavors, progress in caring for a loved one with dementia requires ongoing growth and change. Not only is a loved one a nesting doll, but so are we. Each new phase of change calls us to open ourselves and look within to appreciate the fine details of our own emotions and identity. As we said, we do not have a choice in whether our loved one develops dementia, but we do have choices concerning how we will live out our care partner roles so that we can move toward well-being, consistency, and meaning.

One mastery-related choice that we have tried to make of late is to picture that we are not alone in the rip current of caregiving. Instead, we picture that Mom is there with us in the rip current. As we are all being pulled away from shore, we are firmly holding each other's hands as we're calmly treading water and keeping our eyes on the shore of one another. We are there looking into each other's eyes as we embrace the uncertainty of not knowing when the current will ease up yet trusting that the current is one that we will travel together. Should the time come when it is time to let go of Mom's hand, we trust also that we will continue to hold on to her in our hearts. There in the water, we may have untangled some emotions, but we will forever be knotted more deeply in love.

CHAPTER 13

# Epilogue (Donna)

My mother finished the last lap of her marathon journey with us on July 26, 2024, and finally went home to be with my dad and all their friends. She died peacefully with Tom and me by her side.

While her journey here has ended, for us there will be cooldown laps as we grieve. Some of those laps will be expected and some will be unexpected, but that is a subject for other books. I suspect we will find wisdom, comfort, and guidance in the experience of others, much like we hope this book has provided for you on your journey as a care partner.

We talk a lot in this book about being "in the moment" and looking for the spots of brightness in the journey, seeing the unwavering spark of God within the outwardly changing persona of those we are caring for. We were given testimony to that reality in my mother's final day.

When a resident of my mom's facility passes away, the staff have a beautiful tradition. A special handmade quilt is placed over the body and gurney for the trip out of the building to the funeral home. All the staff who can possibly leave their assignment, whether they are direct care, clinical, administrative, or support, form a two-line honor guard lining the way between the unit where the resident lived and the front door of the building. It is a beautiful way for the staff to show respect, say goodbye, and acknowledge that they are also experiencing the loss of someone who mattered.

The funeral director commented to us that during his time with my mother readying her body and in this goodbye walk, he was struck by how many of the staff gravitated toward her and wanted to say goodbye. He commented that she must have been well loved.

For Tom and me, this was a powerful testament to our experience of Mom as a "nesting doll." My mother lived in this facility for almost five years and had already begun the second half of her marathon with dementia when she moved in. At that point, I remember feeling sad that she was "so different" than she had been, and I recall thinking that the staff would never know her how we had known her. I so wanted people to see and appreciate who she was. I was often so stuck in my mourning for who she no longer was that I failed to notice her care team appreciating and relating to her as she was in the present. While I saw how she was "different," they only saw what they loved.

In her final walk from the building, the staff showed us that they had seen the littlest nesting doll—my mother's core being—and found it beautiful. They provided the final lesson in loving who she was at each moment on her journey without the weight of grieving who she wasn't. It was a beautiful and comforting gift to us and a validation of what we had always believed but couldn't always perceive: Although dementia made it harder to see, it could not strip her of her core and essence as a person.

# Acknowledgments

While each rip current survival step has been important for us as care partners, the most vital component has been "yell for help." In caring for Mom and in publishing this book, we know we could never have done it alone.

In caring for Mom, we are grateful to our family and friends who have been there to support us. Your love, concern, and assistance have been—and continue to be—absolute blessings. We are especially grateful to BJ Raby for all the quality time you spent with Mom and for helping her stay connected to her faith in God.

We have also been blessed by the knowledge and support of many professionals in the field of dementia care, especially Patty O'Brian. Patty has been our support group leader through the Alzheimer's Association of Connecticut and an important resource through the Center for Healthy Aging. In many ways, Patty, you are the head lifeguard on Care Partner Beach.

To our support group members both past and present, we cannot thank you enough for being there with us through all the moments of joy and laughter, sadness and tears, tension and fears, etc. Each of you will always have a special place in our hearts.

We also want to express our deepest thanks and appreciation to the staff of LiveWell, Mom's home for the last five years. The way you strive to care for and affirm the dignity of all in your community is inspirational, and we will never forget the way you always valued Mom as a person.

To the staff of Franciscan Home Care and Hospice Care, thank you for joining the journey of these last months and bringing such comfort to Mom and to our family.

To Corrin Campbell, Director of Navigation at LiveWell, thank you for your feedback on our manuscript and ideas for making it better and a more helpful tool for care partners.

In publishing this book, we are grateful to the team at Greenleaf Book Group for your support and guidance. Your knowledge, creativity, flexibility, and professionalism are amazing. We will also never forget the care, concern, and compassion you have extended to us.

Finally, we are grateful to God for His ever-present guiding hand and role as the ultimate care partner.

APPENDIX

# Care Partner Resources

## Health-Care Support

- Alzheimer's Association Community Resource Finder: https://www.communityresourcefinder.org/
- Eldercare Locator: https://eldercare.acl.gov/Public/Index.aspx
- National Association for Home Care and Hospice: https://nahc.org/
- Medicare Locator for Home Health Services: https://www.medicare.gov/care-compare/?redirect=true&providerType=HomeHealth
- Administration for Community Living Eldercare Locator: https://eldercare.acl.gov/Public/Index.aspx
- Meals on Wheels America: https://www.mealsonwheelsamerica.org/
- National Adult Day Services Association: https://www.nadsa.org/locator/
- National Respite Network and Resource Center: https://archrespite.org/caregiver-resources/respitelocator/

## Legal Guidance

- National Academy of Elder Law Attorneys: https://www.naela.org//

## Telephone Care Partner Support Hotlines

- Alzheimer's Association 24-Hour Helpline: (800-272-3900)
- Alzheimer's Foundation of America Helpline: Phone (866-232-8484), Text (646-586-5283)

## Dementia Education

- Alzheimer's Foundation of America: https://alzfdn.org
- Alzheimer's Association Educational Programs: https://www.alz.org/help-support/resources/care-education-resources
- National Institute on Aging (NIA): https://www.nia.nih.gov/
- National Institutes of Health Alzheimer's Caregiving: https://www.nia.nih.gov/health/alzheimers/caregiving
- U.S. Department of Veterans Affairs VA Caregiver Support Programs: https://www.caregiver.va.gov/

## Care Partner Support Groups

- Alzheimer's Association Support Group Locator: https://www.alz.org/events/event_search?etid=2&cid=0
- ALZCONNECTED (virtual discussion forum): https://alzconnected.org/

# Notes

## Preface

1. Alzheimer's Association, *Alzheimer's Disease Facts and Figures*, 2024, https://www.alz.org/media/Documents/alzheimers-facts-and-figures.pdf.

## Chapter 1

1. Alzheimer's Association, *Alzheimer's Disease Facts and Figures*, 20; World Health Organization, "Dementia: Key Facts," March 15, 2023, https://www.who.int/news-room/fact-sheets/detail/dementia.
2. "What Happens to the Brain in Alzheimer's Disease?," National Institute on Aging, January 19, 2024, https://www.nia.nih.gov/health/alzheimers-causes-and-risk-factors/what-happens-brain-alzheimers-disease.
3. "What Happens to the Brain in Alzheimer's Disease?"
4. Alzheimer's Association, *Alzheimer's Disease Facts and Figures*, 46.
5. Anil Kumar et al., "Stress: Neurobiology, Consequences and Management," *Journal of Pharmacy and Bioallied Sciences* 5, no. 2 (Apr–Jun 2013): 91–97, https://www.ncbi.nlm.nih.gov/pmc/articles/PMC3697199/.
6. Alzheimer's Association, "Take Care of Yourself: How to Recognize and Manage Caregiver Stress," 2018, https://nursing.osu.edu/sites/default/files/attachments/Offices%20and%20Initiatives/FDC/Caregiver-Stress-Topic-Sheet.pdf.

## Chapter 2

1. American Psychiatric Association, *Diagnostic and Statistical Manual of Mental Disorders*, 5th ed. (Washington, DC: American Psychiatric Publishing Inc., 2013), 593–95.
2. Alzheimer's Association, "10 Warning Signs of Alzheimer's," May 2023, https://www.alz.org/media/Documents/alzheimers-dementia-ten_warning-signs-ts.pdf; Nancy Mace and Peter Rabins, *The 36-Hour Day*, 6th ed. (Baltimore: Johns Hopkins University Press, 2017).
3. American Psychiatric Association, *Diagnostic and Statistical*, 602–5.
4. American Psychiatric Association, *Diagnostic and Statistical*, 611–43.
5. Alzheimer's Association, *Alzheimer's Disease Facts and Figures*, 6.
6. American Psychiatric Association, *Diagnostic and Statistical*, 612.
7. American Psychiatric Association, *Diagnostic and Statistical*, 613.
8. American Psychiatric Association, *Diagnostic and Statistical*, 621–22.
9. William McDonald, "Overview of Neurocognitive Disorders," *Focus* 15, no. 1 (Winter 2017), https://psychiatryonline.org/doi/pdf/10.1176/appi.focus.20160030.
10. American Psychiatric Association, *Diagnostic and Statistical*, 614–16.
11. American Psychiatric Association, *Diagnostic and Statistical*, 616.
12. American Psychiatric Association, *Diagnostic and Statistical*, 618–20.
13. American Psychiatric Association, *Diagnostic and Statistical*, 636–37.
14. American Psychiatric Association, *Diagnostic and Statistical*, 642–43.
15. "Delirium," Mayo Clinic, www.mayoclinic.org/diseases-conditions/delirium/symptoms-causes/syc-20371386.

## Chapter 4

1. "Help and Support," Alzheimer's Association, https://www.alz.org/help-support.
2. Eldercare Locator, Administration for Community Living, https://eldercare.acl.gov/Public/Index.aspx.

## Chapter 5

1. National Academy of Elder Law Attorneys, https://www.naela.org//.

## Chapter 6

1. Seth Gillihan, *Cognitive Behavioral Therapy Made Simple: 10 Strategies for Managing Anxiety, Depression, Anger, Panic, and Worry* (Berlin: Callisto Publishing, 2018).
2. Judith Beck, *Cognitive Behavior Therapy: Basics and Beyond*, 3rd ed. (New York: Guilford Press, 2021).
3. Jeffrey Young, Janet Klosko, and Marjorie Weishaar, *Schema Therapy: A Practitioner's Guide* (New York: Guilford Press, 2003).

## Chapter 7

1. Edmund Bourne, *The Anxiety & Phobia Workbook*, 3rd ed. (Oakland, CA: New Harbinger Publications, 2020).
2. Gia Miller and Stephanie Wright, "The 8 Best Apps for Anxiety in 2022," PsychCentral, March 16, 2022, https://psychcentral.com/reviews/apps-for-anxiety#_noHeaderPrefixedContent.
3. Matthew McKay, Martha Davis, and Patrick Fanning, *Thoughts & Feelings: Taking Control of Your Moods and Your Life*, 3rd ed. (Oakland: New Harbinger Publications, 2007).
4. Alexander Lowen, *Bioenergetics: The Revolutionary Therapy That Uses the Language of the Body to Heal the Problems of the Mind* (New York: Penguin Books, 1976); Helen Kennerley, "Cognitive Therapy of Dissociative Symptoms Associated with Trauma," *British Journal of Clinical Psychology* 35, no. 3 (September 1996): 325–40.
5. Ellen Hendriksen, *How to Be Yourself: Quiet Your Inner Critic and Rise Above Social Anxiety* (New York: St. Martin's Press, 2018).
6. "What You Can Do to Meet Physical Activity Requirements," Centers for Disease Control and Prevention, April 16, 2024, https://www.cdc.gov/physical-activity-basics/guidelines/?CDC_AAref_Val=https://www.cdc.gov/physicalactivity/basics/age-chart.html.
7. "About Sleep," Centers for Disease Control and Prevention, https://www.cdc.gov/sleep/about/?CDC_AAref_Val=https://www.cdc.gov/sleep/about_sleep/sleep_hygiene.html.
8. Michael Perlis, *Cognitive Behavioral Treatment of Insomnia: A Session-by-Session Guide* (New York: Springer Publishing, 2006).
9. "How to Have Healthier Meals and Snacks," Centers for Disease Control and Prevention, https://www.cdc.gov/healthy-weight-growth/

healthy-eating/meals-snacks.html?CDC_AAref_Val=https://www.cdc.gov/healthyweight/healthy_eating/index.html.

## Chapter 8

1. Julian Rotter, *Social Learning and Clinical Psychology* (Upper Saddle River, NJ: Prentice-Hall, Inc., 1954).
2. Raymond DiGiuseppe et al., *A Practitioner's Guide to Rational-Emotive Therapy* (New York: Oxford University Press, 1980).
3. DiGiuseppe et al., *A Practitioner's Guide*, 130.
4. Jon Kabat-Zinn et al., "Effectiveness of a Meditation-Based Stress Reduction Program in the Treatment of Anxiety Disorders," *The American Journal of Psychiatry* 149, no. 7 (August 1992): 936–43; Steven Hayes, Kirk Strosahl, and Kelly Wilson, *Acceptance and Commitment Therapy: An Experiential Approach to Behavior Change* (New York: Guilford Press, 1999).
5. Kabat-Zinn et al., "Effectiveness of a Meditation-Based," 936–43.
6. Russ Harris, *ACT Made Simple: An Easy-To-Read Primer on Acceptance and Commitment Therapy*, 2nd ed. (Oakland, CA: New Harbinger Publications, 2019).
7. Jill Stoddard and Niloofar Afari, *The Big Book of ACT Metaphors: A Practitioner's Guide to Experiential Exercises and Metaphors in Acceptance and Commitment Therapy* (Oakland, CA: New Harbinger Publications, 2014).
8. Matthew McKay, Martha Davis, and Patrick Fanning, *Thoughts & Feelings: Taking Control of Your Moods and Your Life*, 3rd ed. (Oakland, CA: New Harbinger Publications, 2007); Glenn Schiraldi, *The Self-Esteem Workbook* (Oakland, CA: New Harbinger Publications, 2001); Steven Hayes and Spencer Smith, *Get out of Your Mind and into Your Life* (Oakland, CA: New Harbinger Publications, 2005).

## Chapter 10

1. Pope John Paul II, "Message of John Paul II on the Occasion of the International Symposium on the Dignity and Rights of the Mentally Disabled Person," International Symposium on the Dignity and Rights of the Mentally Disabled Person, January 5, 2004, Vatican City, Italy, https://www.vatican.va/content/john-paul-ii/en/speeches/2004/january/documents/hf_jp-ii_spe_20040108_handicap-mentale.html.

2. Nathaniel Hawthorne, "The Birth-Mark," in *Mosses from an Old Manse* (London: Wiley and Putnam, 1846).
3. DiGiuseppe et al., *A Practitioner's Guide*, 118–25.
4. Helen Keller, *The Open Door* (Garden City, NY: Doubleday, 1957).
5. J. K. Rowling, *Harry Potter and the Order of the Phoenix* (New York: Bloomsbury Publishing, 2003).

## Chapter 11

1. Marsha Linehan, *Skills Training Manual for Treating Borderline Personality Disorder* (New York: Guilford Press, 1993).
2. "Teddy Roosevelt's Metaphor," *The New York Times Magazine*, print archive, March 9, 1986, https://www.nytimes.com/1986/03/09/magazine/l-teddy-roosevelt-s-metaphor-605086.html.

## Chapter 12

1. Ray Kroc and Robert Anderson, *Grinding It Out: The Making of McDonald's* (New York: St. Martin's Paperbacks, 2016).

# Glossary

**Alzheimer's disease**—Neurocognitive disorder characterized by gradual and increasing declines in memory and ability to learn new information.

**Awfulizing**—The tendency to lose perspective on daily experiences leading to increased stress, which is reflected in thoughts and statements such as *This is awful* or *This is overwhelming*.

**Caregiver**—Term used to describe the people who *give* care to a person with dementia, who *receives* that care in a one-directional relationship. The term risks implication that only the person with dementia is impacted in the giving of care.

**Care partner**—Term used to describe the people involved in a mutual and reciprocal relationship between a person with dementia and the people who provide for their care and support. Each person both gives and receives gifts from the other in ways that foster each other's growth and well-being, both physically and psychologically.

**Care team**—A team of care partners, including professional health-care providers, who provide ongoing services to a person who is experiencing dementia.

**Cognitive behavior therapy (CBT)**—Strategies for emotional and psychological growth and coping drawn from research and experience in the field of cognitive sciences. Such strategies focus on shifting away from self-defeating styles of thinking and behavior to improve health.

**Cognitive domains**—Categories of thinking and other psychologically related skills that include complex attention, executive function, learning and memory, language, perceptual-motor, and social cognition skills.

**Core beliefs/Core fears**—Beliefs about ourself based on messages that we receive through our experiences in life that tell us about the "core" of who we are. Often heard as invalidating "I am" statements, core fears result in pain and fight-or-flight responses when themes of inadequacy, vulnerability, and unimportance are triggered.

**Dementia**—A general term describing problems in brain functioning caused by various underlying conditions, illnesses, and other events that disrupt a person's daily living activities. Symptoms include problems such as memory loss, language deficits, confusion, and other psychological difficulties.

**Dementia with Lewy bodies**—Neurocognitive disorder characterized by bodies of abnormally bunched, or clumped, proteins in the brain that contribute to dementia symptoms, notably problems with sleep and visual hallucinations. Motor difficulties can follow cognitive declines.

**Dignity**—The intrinsic worth that is possessed by each person, which deserves to be universally respected. Dignity reflects the right to be loved and understood and is not earned; it is simply present within each person.

**Frontotemporal lobe dementia**—Neurocognitive disorder characterized by deteriorations in the frontal lobe and temporal lobe of the brain.

**Identity independence**—The recognition that a person's identity, worth, and dignity are not defined by experiences.

**Lack List**—A list of reasons many care partners give for being unable to engage in self-care behaviors like exercise, healthy eating, etc. Reasons can include a lack of time, money, energy, enjoyment, knowledge, and opportunity.

**Locus of control**—A person's view of circumstances being caused either by forces outside of one's control (external locus of control) or by forces within one's control (internal locus of control).

**Low-tolerance thinking**—Thoughts reflecting a belief that one is incapable of coping with the stress of a given situation, such as *I can't stand this anymore* or *I can't take this.*

**Mild cognitive impairment**—Small changes in memory, thinking skills, etc., that do not interfere with daily activities.

**Mindfulness**—Being aware of one's internal and external experiences in each moment, which include noticing and accepting one's thoughts, feelings, and body reactions without judgment, then choosing to act in ways one believes are important.

**Neurocognitive disorders**—A diagnostic classification that encompasses varied symptoms of dementia that have a negative impact on a person's ability to function cognitively, emotionally, behaviorally, and socially.

Specific categories are named after the specific causes of those symptoms and include categories such as Alzheimer's disease and vascular dementia.

**Opposite action**—Recognizing when a feeling is not helpful to a situation and doing the opposite of what that feeling "tells" us to do.

**Resiliency principle**—Knowledge that care partner stress can be borne more productively when one finds a deeper meaning in the struggles and suffering that naturally come when caring for someone with dementia.

**Rip current**—A phenomenon that occurs along ocean coastlines where an alley of water moves away from the beach and out to sea. Sometimes, the power and speed of this outward-bound water can pull a swimmer quickly away from the safety of the shore.

**Self-esteem**—One's opinion of one's self-worth. Self-esteem can change and be measured. Recognition that one's self-worth, dignity, value, and significance as a person cannot be changed by circumstances or experiences.

**Self-worth**—The essence of a person's goodness, competence, and dignity as a human person, which is unchanging and immeasurable.

**Self-worth rating**—Believing that one's worth, value, and dignity as a person can change based on circumstances or experiences.

**Vascular dementia**—Neurocognitive disorder marked by declines in cognitive domains related to problems in blood flow through the brain, often in the form of strokes, ministrokes (temporary ischemic attacks, or TIAs), stenosis of the carotid arteries, cerebral aneurysms, etc.

# Index

## A

acting opposite, 133–37
advance directives, 44
    DNR/DNI orders, 45
Administration for Community Living Eldercare Locator, 36, 38, 173
Alzheimer's Association, x, 10, 36, 111–14,
    24 Hour Helpline, 174
    ALZCONNECTED online discussion forum, 114, 174
    Community Resource Finder, 36, 173
    stress management guidelines, 10–11
ALZCONNECTED online discussion forum, 114, 174
Alzheimer's disease, viii, 23–24, 181
Alzheimer's Foundation of America, 112, 173
    Helpline, 174
anchoring (grounding) tools, 60–61, 97
aphasia, 19
awfulizing, 79–82, 181

## B

behavioral tools for managing stress, 133–63
    changing the subject, 159–63
    communication strategies, 148–51
    connection vs. correction, 147–48
    creative calming, 151–54
    focusing on long-term memory, 140, 161
    greeting when meet, 141
    interaction strategies, 144–46
    limiting distraction, 145–46
    listening, 154–55
        and reflecting emotions, 155–56
        for emotions, 154–56
    opposite action, 136–37
    reassurance, providing, 157–59
    responding to memory issues, 137–40
    staying in the moment, 141–44
biomarkers, 2–3
Beck, Dr. Judith, 51
"Birth-Mark, The," 120–21
brain structure, 25
breathing, gentle, 59–60
    apps for, 60, 177

## C

care decisions, 35–38
caregiver, xi–xii, 181
   education, 112–13, 174
   and stress, 4–11
caregiver support continuum, 108–14
   family support, 109–10
   friends, 110–11
   mental health counseling, 114
   online forums, 113
   phone hotlines, 112, 174
   primary care physicians, 111
   support agencies, 111
   support groups, 113
caregiver vs. care partner, terminology, xi–xii
care partner, xi–xii, 181
care team, 35–38
CBT-I, 67
Center for Healthy Aging, 20, 113
changing the subject, 159–63
cognitive behavioral perspective, 50
cognitive behavior therapy (CBT), 72, 182
CBT (cognitive behavior therapy), 72, 182
cognitive behavior therapy for insomnia, 67
cognitive domains, 17–20, 182
   complex attention, 17
   executive functions, 17
   language, 18
   learning and memory, 17
   perceptual motor, 18
   social cognition, 18
cognitive tests, 32–33
competence, 87
complex attention, 17, 18
   as cognitive domain, 17
   as dementia symptom, 18
communication strategies, 148–51
connection vs. correction, 147–48
conservator, 45–46
coping, physical, 57–69
core beliefs, 50–52, 84–85, 182
   and stress exercise, 53–54
   as triggers in care partner relationships, 51–54
   shifting, 91–95
creative calming, 151–54

## D

defusion strategies, 98
delirium, 27–28
dementia, x–xi, 21–22, 182
   statistics, 1
   symptoms of, 17–21
   subtypes, 22–27
      dementia due to
         Alzheimer's disease, 23–24
         frontotemporal lobe degeneration, 25–26, 183
         lewy bodies, 26, 182
         other causes, 27
         Parkinson's dementia, 26–27
         vascular disease, 24–25
"Dementia Crisis," global, 1
dementia, mixed, 27
dementia due to multiple etiologies, 27
DNR/DNI orders, 45
diet and nutrition (in managing stress), 68–69
   healthy eating guidelines, 68, 177–78
dignity, 9, 87, 118–19, 182
dimensions of personhood, 5–6
disrupted equilibrium, 5, 120
Doleski, Teddi, 78

## E

education for caregivers, 112–13
Eldercare Locator, 36, 173
emotional development, 50–52
emotional relationship with loved ones, 49
emotional triggers, 52–54
emotional vocabulary exercise, 76–77
emotions, 74–78
   exploring, 156–57
   listening for, 154–55
   reflecting, 155–56
equilibrium, disrupted, 5, 120

essence, human, 86
estate planning, 40–46
Every Time is the First Time, principle of, 137–39
executive functions, 17–19
    as cognitive domain, 17–18
    as dementia symptom, 18–19
exercise, 62–64

## F

family, support from, 109–10
feelings, 74–78
    exploring, 156–57
    listening for, 154–55
    reflecting, 155–56
feelings vocabulary exercise, 76–77
feelings vs. thinking, 72–76
fight-or-flight response, 6–9, 57–58
financial planning, 40–41, 46–47
friends, support from, 110–11
frontotemporal lobe dementia, 25–26, 183

## G

genetic tests, 34
geriatric nurse practitioner, 31
geriatric psychiatrist, 31
geriatrician, 31
gerontologist, 31
global "Dementia Crisis," 1
goodness, human, 86–87
geropsychologist, 31
greet when meet, 141
grief, 9, 114, 121, 126
grounding strategies, sensory (anchoring), 60–61, 97
guardian, 45–46

## H

Hawthorne, Nathaniel, 120
health care agent, 44
Hendrickson, Dr. Ellen, 61
*Hurt, The*, 78

## I

*I Love Lucy*, 148
identity independence, 91–95, 183
identity independence exercise, 92–94
    in accepting support, 106–8
information processing, in dementia, 142–44
interaction strategies, 144–46

## J

John Paul II, Pope, 119

## K

Keller, Helen, 126

## L

laboratory tests, 33
Lack List, 63–64, 68, 183
language, 18, 19
    as cognitive domain 18
    as dementia symptom, 19
last will and testament, 42
learning and memory, 17, 19
    as cognitive domain, 17
    as dementia symptom, 19
legal planning, 42–46, 174
lewy bodies, dementia with, 26, 182
limiting distraction, 145–46
listening, 154–55
    for emotions, 154–56
    and reflecting emotions, 155–56
Linehan, Dr. Marsha, 136
Listen, Reassure, and Change the Subject, principle of, 154–83
locus of control, 72–74, 182
    external, 72
    internal, 73
long-term memory, focusing on 140, 161
love, 130–32
    deepening, 130–31
    witnessing to, 131–32

low-tolerance thinking, 82–84, 183

## M

mastery of stress, ix–x
Meals on Wheels America, 38, 173
Medicare Home Health Services Locator, 38, 173
memory, 17, 19, 137–41
    as cognitive domain, 17
    as dementia symptom, 19
    responding to memory problems, 137–41
mental health counseling, 114
mental health tests, 34
metaphors, visual, 98–99
mild cognitive impairment (MCI), 21–22, 183
mindfulness, 95–101, 127–28, 141–42, 183
    defusion strategies, 98
    NAC exercise, 98
    visual imagery/metaphors, 98–99
mixed dementia, 23, 27

## N

NAC mindfulness exercise, 98
National Academy of Elder Law Attorneys, 174

perceptual motor skills, 18, 19
    as cognitive domain, 18
    as dementia symptom, 19
personhood, 5–6
phone calls (nighttime), 66–67, 96–97
phone hotlines, 112, 174
physical movement in managing stress, 62–64
physical tools for managing stress, 58–69
    breathing, gentle, 59–60
        apps for, 60, 177
    diet and nutrition, 68–69

National Adult Day Services Association, 38, 173
National Association of Home Care and Hospice, 37, 111, 173
National Institutes of Health Alzheimer's Caregiving, 174
National Institutes on Aging, 174
National Respite Network Resource Center, 38, 173
nesting doll analogy, 167
neurocognitive disorders, x–xi, 21–22, 183
    mild, 21
    major, 21
    subtypes, 22–28
neurological tests, 33–34
neurologist, 32
neuropsychologist, 32
nighttime phone calls, 66–67, 96–97
nutrition and diet, 68–69
    healthy guidelines for, 68, 177–78

## O

online support forums, 113, 174
*Open Door, The*, 126
opposite action, 136–37, 184

## P

Parkinson's dementia, 26–27

exercise, 62–64
physical movement, 62–64
sensory grounding tools, 60–61, 97
sleep, 65–67
    cognitive behavioral treatment for insomnia (CBT-I), 67
    phone calls (nighttime), 66–67, 96–97
    sleep hygiene, 65–66
psychological tools for managing stress, 78–101
    de-awfulized thinking, 79–82

# Index

discomfort tolerance thinking, 82–84
identity independence, 91–95
mindfulness, 95–101, 127–28, 141–42
   defusion strategies, 98
   NAC exercise, 98
   visual imagery/metaphors, 98–99
preference thinking, 122–24
realistic thinking, 78–79
self-acceptance, 85–86, 105–8
WHATIFIO, 100–101
Pope John Paul II, 119
power of attorney, 43
*Practitioner's Guide to Rational-Emotive Therapy*, 79
preference thinking, 122–24
preparing for primary care physician appointments, 30–31
present, simplicity in, 127–28
primary care physicians (PCP), 29–30, 111
   as support, 111
   preparation for appointments with, 30–31

## R

reassurance, providing, 157–59
relationship patterns with loved ones, 49–54
Resiliency Principle, 78, 184
resources for care, 36–38, 173–74
responding to memory issues, 137–40
rip current, 11–12, 57, 184
   surviving, 12–13
Roosevelt, Theodore, 139
Rowling, J. K., 127

## S

self-acceptance, 85–86
   in asking for help, 105–8
self-care, 11

self-esteem, 88–91, 184
self-worth, 86–88, 184
self-worth rating, 84–85, 184
self-worth vs. self-esteem, 86–91
sensory grounding tools, 60–61, 97
should statements, 122–24
simplicity, 127–28
sleep, 65–67
   cognitive behavior therapy for insomnia, 67
   phone calls (nighttime), 66–67, 96–97
   sleep hygiene, 65–66
social cognition, 18, 20
   as cognitive domain, 18
   as dementia symptom, 20
social support, 103–4
staying in the moment, 141–44
stress, 4–5, 6–11, 57–58, 120–22
   causes of, 4
   defined, 5–7
   fight-or-flight response, 6–7
   impacts of, 7–11
      emotional, 8–9
      physical, 8
      social, 9
      spiritual, 10
   mastery of, defined, ix
stress management, 10–11
   behavioral tools for, 133–63
      changing the subject, 159–63
      communication strategies, 148–51
      connection vs. correction, 147–48
      creative calming, 151–54
      focusing on long-term memory, 140, 161
      greeting when meet, 141
      interaction strategies, 144–46
      limiting distraction, 145–46
      listening, 154–55
         and reflecting emotions, 155–56
         for emotions, 154–56
      opposite action, 136–37
      reassurance, providing, 157–59

responding to memory issues, 137–40
staying in the moment, 141–44
physical tools for, 58–69
  breathing, gentle, 59–60
    apps for, 60, 177
  diet and nutrition, 68–69
  exercise, 62–64
  physical movement, 62–64
  sensory grounding tools, 60–61, 97
  sleep, 65–67
    cognitive behavioral treatment for insomnia (CBT-I), 67
    phone calls (nighttime), 66–67, 96–97
    sleep hygiene, 65–66
psychological tools for, 78–101
  de-awfulized thinking, 79–82
  discomfort tolerance thinking, 82–84
  identity independence, 91–95
  mindfulness, 95–101, 127–28, 141–42
    defusion strategies, 98
    NAC exercise, 98
    visual imagery/metaphors, 98–99
  preference thinking, 122–24
  realistic thinking, 78–79
  self-acceptance, 85–86, 105–8
  WHATIFIO, 100–101
suffering, transformation through, 126–27
support
  accepting, 105–8
  agencies for, 111–12, 174
  avoiding, 104–5
  caregiver support continuum, 108–14
    family support, 109–10
    friends, 110–11
    mental health counseling, 114
    online forums, 113
    phone hotlines, 112, 174
    primary care physicians, 111
    support agencies, 111

    support groups, 113
  care team, 35–38
  groups, 113, 174
support agencies, 111–12, 173
support groups, 113, 174
support group locator, 114
symptoms of dementia, 17–28

## T

tests, 32–34
  cognitive, 32–33
  genetic, 34
  laboratory, 33
  mental health, 34
  neurological, 33–34
The Only Moment is This Moment, principle of, 141–54
  defined, 141–42
"The Birth-Mark," 120–21
*The Hurt*, 78
*The Open Door*, 126
thinking, 73, 74–85, 122–24
  awfulizing, 79–82
  low-tolerance thinking, 82–84
  realistic, 78–79
  preference, 122–24
  self-worth rating, 84–85
  should statements, 122–24
  unrealistic, 79
  vs. feeling, 72–76
  what if, 100
Thestral beasts, 127

## U

unfairness, 121–22
  and lack of family support, 125
unrealistic thinking, 79
U.S. Department of Veterans Affairs VA Caregiver Support, 174

## V

values vs. good ideas, 63–64
vascular disease, dementia due to, 23, 24–25, 184
visual imagery, 98–99

## W

WHATIFIO, 100
wisdom of threes (sensory grounding strategy), 60–61
what if thinking, 100
Who Am I exercise, 92–94
   in accepting support, 106–8

## Y

Young, Dr. Jeffrey, 50–51

# About the Authors

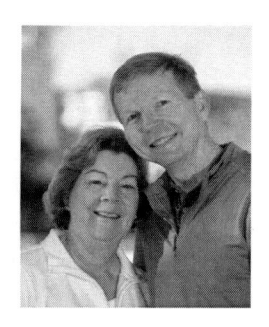

The Finns live in Southington, Connecticut, and have three children, two sons-in-law, a daughter-in-law, and five grandchildren. Together, the Finns have led workshops and retreats on topics of mastering caregiving stress, marriage enrichment, communication, and team building for adults, children, families, and organizations.

Thomas Finn, PhD, has worked for forty years as a clinical psychologist in a variety of settings and is currently on the staff of the Franciscan Life Center in Meriden, Connecticut. With expertise in the application of cognitive behavior therapy for anxiety and stress, he has also led seminars on anxiety, relationships, pastoral counseling, and organizational development in the US and abroad. He received his master's and doctorate degrees in clinical-school psychology from Hofstra University and a bachelor of arts degree in psychology from Fairfield University.

Donna M. Finn, PT, MS, has worked as a physical therapist for over forty years, serving in leadership positions in many health-care settings, including Yale New Haven Hospital, Franciscan Home Care and Hospice Care, and Hartford HealthCare at Home. She holds a master of science degree in health sciences administration from the State University of New York at Stony Brook, a professional certificate in physical therapy from Columbia University, and a bachelor of science degree in biology from Fairfield University.

Made in United States
North Haven, CT
30 March 2025